Moral Laboratories

The publisher gratefully acknowledges the generous support of the General Endowment Fund of the University of California Press Foundation.

Moral Laboratories

*Family Peril and the Struggle for
a Good Life*

Cheryl Mattingly

UNIVERSITY OF CALIFORNIA PRESS

University of California Press, one of the most
distinguished university presses in the United States,
enriches lives around the world by advancing scholarship
in the humanities, social sciences, and natural sciences. Its
activities are supported by the UC Press Foundation and
by philanthropic contributions from individuals and
institutions. For more information, visit www.ucpress.edu.

University of California Press
Oakland, California

Library of Congress Cataloging-in-Publication Data

Mattingly, Cheryl, 1951-
  Moral laboratories : family peril and the struggle for a
good life / Cheryl Mattingly.
      p.   cm.
  Includes bibliographical references and index.
  ISBN 978-0-520-28119-6 (hardback)
  ISBN 978-0-520-28120-2 (paper)
  ISBN 978-0-520-95953-8 (e-book)
  1. Chronically ill children—Medical care—Moral and
ethical aspects—California—Los Angeles County.   2.
Children with disabilities—Medical care—Moral and
ethical aspects—California—Los Angeles County.   3.
African American families—California—Los Angeles
County.   4. Medical anthropology—California—Los
Angeles County.   5. Medical ethics—California—Los
Angeles County.   I. Title.
  RJ380.M28 2014
  362.19892009794 93—dc23   2014006568

23   22   21   20   19   18   17   16   15   14
10   9   8   7   6   5   4   3   2   1

To Steven, again

Contents

Acknowledgments

This is the second book to emerge from an ethnographic project that has followed African American families and their children in the Los Angeles area. It represents nearly fifteen years of research and the efforts of many people. It has grown out of the work of many partners over the years, including colleagues, former students, and friends. Mary Lawlor, my long-term research partner, is the most important person to mention. Together, we have served as principal and coprincipal investigators on a series of grants that have funded this research. Mary's insights into the moral struggles that families face have continued to influence my own thoughts. Lanita Jacobs, a linguistic anthropologist, joined our team as a coinvestigator in 1999. The nuanced way she speaks and writes about race, her own first person perspective on how it is lived, have continued to haunt my thinking.

Then there are the many researchers, graduate students, postdoctoral fellows, and research faculty who have spent some years on the project. Not only have these colleagues been an essential part of ethnographic fieldwork, they have also contributed numerous conceptual insights over the years through our "data interpretation" groups. Although no one has been involved for the duration of the project except Mary and me, many were part of it for three years or more, reflecting shifts in our funding and people's personal lives. Core researchers have been Jeanne Adams, Kim Wilkinson, Nancy Bagatelle, Kevin Groark, Olga Solomon, Melissa Park, Teresa Kuan, Nancy Bagatelle, Erica

Angert, Carolyn Rouse, Alice Kibele, Janine Blanchard, and Courtney Mykytyn. Several other colleagues have been part of the data analysis or have substantially contributed to other forms of research support (literature reviews and the like) that I have benefited from directly. These include Katy Sanders, Juleon Rabbani, Anita Kumar, Teresa Kuan, Melissa Park, Jason Throop, Aaron Bonsall, Michelle Elliot, Daylan Riggs, Cynthia Strathman, and Lindsay Miller. But there are many others who have worked on this study over the years, graduate and undergraduate students at the University of Southern California who have supported this research in invaluable ways: transcribing interviews and videotapes of clinic and home sessions, videotaping the Collective Narrative Groups, providing computer support, or taking care of children while parents talked to the research team. Although I can't name them all here, I offer a heartfelt thanks to this dedicated crew.

And then there are the readers, people inside and outside the project who have read various versions of this book manuscript over the years. They have helped me see what I was saying when I myself was unclear. This is another long list. The most central are friends as well as colleagues: Mary Lawlor, Lone Grøn, Melissa Park, Teresa Kuan, and Lotte Meinert and Uffe Juul Jensen. They have played special roles over the years as a friends and sympathetic challengers, asking me essential and critical questions from their own philosophical positions. Finally, there are the readers who helped me to shape the book in the end. These include Art Frank and Jason Throop, reviewers whose comments and suggestions were so apt that they made the daunting task of revision more bearable. Reed Malcolm, University of California Press editor, has played a crucial role in helping to move this book along.

None of the chapters in this book, as they now stand, has appeared anywhere else in print. However, versions of some of the cases, and bits and pieces of previously published work, have been integrated within these book chapters. (Often I have changed pseudonyms in various publications to help protect the confidentiality of research participants.) Earlier published work in which some materials from this book have appeared includes: "Love's Imperfection: Moral Becoming, Friendship and Family Life" (Mattingly [in press]), "The Moral Perils of a Superstrong Black Mother" (Mattingly 2014), "What Can We Hope For? An Exploration in Cosmopolitan Philosophical Anthropology" (Mattingly and Jensen [in press]), "Moral Selves and Moral Scenes: Narrative Experiments in Everyday Life" (Mattingly 2013), "Two Virtue Ethics and the Anthropology of Morality" (Mattingly 2012), "The Machine

Body as Contested Metaphor in Clinical Care" (Mattingly 2011), "I/We Narratives among African American Families Raising Children with Disabilities" (Jacobs, Lawlor, and Mattingly 2011), "Chronic Homework in Emerging Borderlands of Healthcare" (Mattingly, Grøn, and Meinert, 2011), "Reading Medicine: Mind, Body, and Meditation in One Interpretive Community" (Mattingly 2006a), and "Suffering and Narrative Re-envisioning" (Mattingly 2006b).

I have presented earlier versions of some of these chapters—or parts of them—in many places and to a range of academic and clinical groups, both in the United States and in Europe, especially Denmark. Such presentations, and the discussions they have engendered from the audience, have helped immeasurably in the formulation of my arguments. Although I could give a long list of conferences, I single out several communities that, at different times, have played the most significant role— outside the research team, of course—in providing me a space to think things through.

One is a community of Danish researchers, primarily in anthropology and philosophy, at the University of Aarhus. The Center for Health, Humanity and Culture, Department of Philosophy and History of Ideas, under the direction of Uffe Juul Jensen, has offered a crucial intellectual home, even when visits have been sporadic. In the fall of 2009, a joint guest professorship in the Department of Philosophy and the History of Ideas and the Department of Anthropology and Ethnography at the University of Aarhus provided financial support and an invaluable source of discussions as I revised the book manuscript—especially chapter 2. More recently, a Danish group of philosophers and anthropologists, especially Thomas Wentzer and Rasmus Dyring, interested in developing a new kind of philosophical anthropology focusing upon the phenomenology of morality, has contributed enormously to my thinking. The work on this book could not have been completed without the support of the Division of Occupational Science under Dr. Florence Clark, and the Dale T. Mortensen research fellowship I have received from Aarhus University's Institute of Advanced Studies under Professor Morten Kyndrup. In one sense, this book is also part of a future that will continue to involve collaborations with colleagues associated with the Institute and Aarhus University.

A second is the Mind, Medicine, and Culture Seminar, a space where a group of medical, psychological, and linguistic anthropologists at the University of California, Los Angeles, regularly talk. I have presented to this seminar on occasion and attended when I could. Several members of this group, graduate students and faculty, have read earlier versions of various manuscripts that have (in some form or another) found their way into chapters in this book. This seminar has been one place that has fostered scholars interested in cultivating person-centered and phenomenological perspectives in their anthropological fieldwork and theorizing.

Though it has been some years since we got together, a third community I mention is one that Linda Garro and I organized—we called it the Narrative Group. Anthropology faculty from both the University of Southern California and University of California, Los Angeles with wide-ranging interests in narrative met about once a month to discuss working papers. Participants were Candy Goodwin, Janet Hoskins, Nancy Lutkehaus, Geyla Frank, Mary Lawlor, and Elinor Ochs.

My husband, Steven Heth, deserves special mention, not only as a source of support and as a listener to half-formed ideas, but for helping me in all kinds of practical ways, including his inspired idea for the cover art. It is difficult to convey how much his presence has meant in my life or how deeply it has influenced my understanding of the ethics of care, commitment and love that is also friendship.

I step back in time to thank some communities and individuals who have played such a vital role in shaping my work on narrative and the phenomenology of illness and healing. A Harvard group of medical anthropologists (funded for many years by the National Institutes of Mental Health), under the direction of Arthur Kleinman, Mary-Jo DelVecchio Good, and Byron Good, offered me a first entrance into the world of medical anthropology. Glenn Bidwell and I had conversations in philosophy thirty years ago that, in a number of ways, provided a beginning for the ideas I continue to develop and write about here.

This ethnographic study has been made possible by several major federally funded grants, and I acknowledge them here: (1) "Crossing Cultural Boundaries: An Ethnographic Study," funded from 1997 to 1999 by Maternal and Child Health in the Department of Health and Human Services; (2) "Boundary Crossing: An Ethnographic and Longitudinal Study," funded from 2000 to 2004 (#1 R01-HD38878) by National Center for Medical Rehabilitation Research in the National Institute of Child Health and Human Development, National Institutes of Health; and (3) "Boundary Crossings: RE-Situating Cultural Competence," funded from 2005 to 2011 (#2 R01-HD38878), again by the National Center for Medical Rehabilitation Research in the National Institute of Child Health and Human Development, National Institutes of Health. The National Institutes of Health also provided supplemental grants that supported two vital members of the research team: Lanita Jacobs (#3 R01 HD38878–01A1S1) and Ann Neville-Jan. Additional support has been provided over the years by the Division of Occupational Science and Occupational Therapy under the direction of Dr. Florence Clark.

The artist, Maggie Michaels, has graciously allowed me to use one of her wonderful works for my cover art. I thank her as well.

Finally, I thank the many clinicians, children, and family members who have allowed us such access to their lives. There has been such generosity. People have given time, a willingness to speak frankly, often about difficult matters, and—in the case of families—invitations to all manner of family events. I have never carried out research where people invited me in to this extent. It would not have been possible for me to write this kind of book, to tackle the questions I do, without such openness. Although, to protect confidentiality I cannot name them personally, I hope that my gratitude can be heard.

Prologue

Once in the late 1980s (more or less), when I was still an unsure graduate student, I attended a panel at one of the annual American Anthropology Association meetings. It was one of those panels whose audience
fills an entire hotel conference ballroom. I've long since forgotten the
topic. The important thing was that extremely influential scholars from
both anthropology and philosophy spoke on the panel. Two of my
favorite philosophers were there—Charles Taylor and Hubert Dreyfus.
They each discussed Heidegger and the significance of his phenomenology for anthropology. They amicably referred to one another's work in
their talks. I was no expert, but I had read both Dreyfus and Taylor on
Heidegger and it seemed to me they should be disagreeing. I had also
been to various philosophy conferences in the past and had heard philosophers in heated debate. I knew they liked to be contentious, and I'd
always found this very educational. (I had once scrounged money early
in my graduate career to attend a critical theory conference in
Dubrovnik—in what was then Yugoslavia—where Gadamer and Habermas were promised to debate.)

But at this anthropology panel, there sat Dreyfus and Taylor chatting
agreeably with one another on stage. I was puzzled. Finally, near the
very end of the session, just as Dreyfus, led by Paul Rabinow, left the
conference table and was heading down the aisle wheeling his suitcase,
I screwed up my courage to stand up and ask a question. "I know you
have to leave, Professor Dreyfus," I ventured timidly, nodding in his

departing direction and then turning to face Taylor, still on stage. "But as I have read both of you, it has seemed to me that you each have very different interpretations of Heidegger's phenomenology. Have I got that wrong?" Dreyfus broke into a great grin, turned around and energetically wheeled his suitcase back toward the stage. Rabinow followed him in surprise. "You are absolutely right," he said, returning to his seat. Taylor nodded. And the two of them spent another fifteen minutes or so defending their versions of Heidegger in cheerful dispute.

Their conversation has stayed with me not only because I admired their fondness for discussion but also because I was trying to understand how to think with phenomenology. I could see that one approach tended to focus on practices themselves. This seemed to me what Dreyfus was most concerned with. His Heidegger offered new ways to consider our practical understandings and activities in phenomenological terms, experientially, as an immersion in the world through our engagement with it. Taylor especially took from Heidegger a way to consider human life, even individual selves. He was drawing from Heidegger's phenomenology of temporality because Taylor was interested in moral becoming from an experiential perspective.

There were obvious overlaps between these two Heideggers, but there was also something not only different, but vitally different, in their approaches. All these years later, I would now put it this way. Taylor was committed to a "thick" first person phenomenology of action, motive, intention, and moral evaluation. Dreyfus was not. His focal concern was practice itself—no strong first person claims of the sort Taylor was advancing were necessary to his phenomenological inquiry. My own moral framework outlined in this book follows Taylor's line of thought much more closely than Dreyfus's. This difference, though apparently subtle, is worth exploring ethnographically as well as theoretically. Or so it seems to me. I also tell this story because this book is filled with debate. In fact, I have never written something so frankly fractious. I write about African American families facing peril, often on many fronts. They are raising children who are seriously, sometimes desperately, ill or disabled. They are very often poor. Many live in dangerous neighborhoods and are presented with an onslaught of disasters. And yet I insist upon an anthropology of morality grounded in a first person virtue ethics that takes disempowered people's moral projects and their beliefs about the good seriously. I do so in a way that regularly puts me at odds with some of the most influential contemporary trends in social theory. I speak of individuals more than about social groups and social categories, the singularities of experience more than its reproductive features, inner emotion and selfhood more often than public personhood. I am primarily concerned with moral possibility and, sometimes, revolutionary transformation, but I rarely explore these in the context of large-scale historical events or transgressive social movements. Rather, I direct my gaze to the humbler moments of everyday life among people who are primarily trying to get by and make do with the (mostly bad) lot that has been handed them. I offer mundane moments of family life as high drama. I look at what seems from an outside (read: middle-class) perspective, like an extraordinary event (a murder, an incarceration), as part of ordinary life. I look at how extraordinary body treacheries (a young child's rare form of brain cancer) are folded into the everyday. Sometimes I catalogue the kinds of social oppression visited upon people, but even here, I attend more to how they creatively and stoically respond to unjust or otherwise miserable social forces than to their underlying causes.

In trying to clear a path for a first person virtue ethics I have admittedly often taken a more contentious route than might seem necessary. Where I might find points of connection, I have often stressed points of disagreement. Where I might have relied upon conciliatory voices, I have opted to highlight those most opinionated and articulate about exactly the points with which I disagree. I hope putting them into debate is of some value, heuristically. I have always preferred a good intellectual fight for its clarifying qualities, though I have tended to prefer it from a seat in the audience. The positions and scholars I have challenged are ones I deeply respect, representing theoretical points of view of great merit that deserve to be taken seriously. They have commanded attention in the academy for good reason. Foucault and what can loosely be called the "Foucauldian tradition" serve as my favored adversaries. Foucault's legacy is of monumental importance. It's fair to say that he has radically altered the way we now think about the workings of institutional and neoliberal power. Certainly he is the single most influential twentieth-century philosopher in anthropology, and his late works on ethics constitute the most significant voice shaping the new anthropology of morality. He—and some scholars inspired by him—are good to think with, and also, at times, good to argue with. In one sense, my debating style throughout reflects an ongoing and troubled love affair with Foucault. His genius has shone such a brilliant light on things that matter a great deal to my own work, including suffering and ethics, that alternative perspectives can be hard to discern, cast as they are into the gloom.

The stories I tell have emerged from many years of research among African American families in Los Angeles. This book has a partner, a work that came out in 2010 (*The Paradox of Hope*) and is also based upon this long-term research. I return to some of the same families that I first introduced in *The Paradox of Hope*. I say less here than perhaps I could have about the research process and the many researchers who have been part of it. For those who would like more details, I refer them to the earlier work.

Although *Moral Laboratories* is not fashionably pessimistic or deconstructive, it is not very optimistic either. If it suffers from a certain Job-like bleakness, this is not only because so many bad things happen to those I write about but also because I treat the idea of miracles with great respect. The people I describe are struggling for good lives against the odds. Even just "getting by" can mean fighting to bring about something new, what Arendt has called the "miracle of natality." This kind of striving is short on happy endings, though it is not short on suspense.

First Person Virtue Ethics

CHAPTER I

Experimental Soccer and the Good Life

THE SOCCER GAME

It could be one of a thousand soccer fields scattered throughout the United States. Grade-school children in their uniforms running up and down the grass shouting to one another as parents cheer them on. An ordinary Saturday afternoon event repeated in countless American towns. Except that in the center of this field, surrounded by screaming children who fly by him, is a boy in a wheelchair propelled by another boy, and they, too, head in the direction of the ball. The boy's father and mother stand at the sidelines watching the action. Tanya and Frank have three children, two girls and a boy who is their oldest. Their son Andy was born with cerebral palsy, an extremely severe case that not only leaves him physically disabled but very cognitively impaired as well. Despite this, Tanya especially knows how to communicate with him and reads his expressions easily. In fact, he shows his temper in no uncertain terms—smiling or glowering with an intensity that is hard to ignore. Tanya is determined to fight for her son's rights to good schooling, and she is fierce in her determination to stand up to school board members, principals, and other public officials to try to get good care for her son. "It's my Jamaican blood," she laughs in justifying her willingness to battle authorities.

But it was her husband Frank who she credits with opening her eyes about her son's capabilities to participate in everyday children's activities that she would have shielded him from. Her husband is an athlete. When the economy was better, he was a personal trainer at a gym, and he is a natural at many sports. A son, his son, should love sports as much as he does, he maintained. Even when Andy was quite young, Frank devised a host of creative ways to bring him into favorite family sports played with his two younger sisters. He installed a basketball hoop in the backyard, and he and Andy would "shoot hoops" together as he lifted him out of the wheelchair high enough above the rim so that Andy could drop the ball and score a goal.

When Andy got older and bigger, Frank decided that he should get Andy involved in the local children's soccer team. Although it was a "special needs" soccer team, the children had cognitive disabilities rather than physical ones. Certainly none used wheelchairs or had the physical frailties Andy did. Tanya was terrified and absolutely refused. She and her husband fought about this for several years. What if he falls? she worried. Soccer can be a rough sport. He is so medically fragile—what can he do in his wheelchair? But her husband prevailed and she let her son go on the field. During one of those games, just as she feared, children accidentally knocked over his wheelchair and he toppled down. But, to her great surprise, he was not only okay; he didn't even seem to mind. He didn't act frightened at all. "Oh I was scared to death," she recounts. "But I guess my husband was right. I didn't realize I was holding Andy back, not letting him be the kid he should get to be." This is a story she has told more than once. It moves her every time. It catches her up short, this realization that despite all her determination that others see her son as capable, she herself underestimated him.

CARE AND ITS MORAL COMPLEXITIES

How might we think of Tanya's situation as an *ethical* problem? How, more specifically, does it pose a problem for her as related to her practices of care? Tanya is one of the parents I have come to know through the years as my colleagues and I have carried out an ethnographic study of African American families in Los Angeles who are raising children with severe disabilities and chronic illnesses. Parents are called upon to try to ascertain what is best for their children and for themselves in the changing circumstances of everyday life and in midst of the many other tasks and problems that they must simultaneously address. This is, in other words, a complex reasoning task that engenders ongoing moral deliberations, evaluations, and experiments in how to live.

In the face of the suffering and challenges of their children, parents often find themselves propelled in a quest to imagine a new sort of life for themselves or to become different kinds of persons. They are propelled into a new, often unexpected and unwanted project of becoming. Suffering can engender new or intensified *moral* responsibilities. These, too, may demand a transformative effort to reimagine not only what will happen, but also what ought to happen, or how one ought to respond not only to difficulties and suffering but also to unexpected possibilities (Mattingly 2010a). The work of care, in other words, demands the work of cultivating virtues to be, for example, a "good enough" parent. As one father put it, you have to "step up to the plate" to raise a very sick child, and this can prove an almost impossible feat. Parents' ability to respond to the call or needs of their vulnerable children, and to create a social world in which their children can be better cared for, become primary moral projects, often superseding their own personal dreams and goals. Furthermore, these are social moral projects that change shape over time, requiring the development of *communities of care,* an expanding "we" that brings together an array of people outside the immediate family, including neighbors and friends, other parents, and clinical professionals.

Such moral work can provoke a critical examination of one's life and one's character, an attempt to transform the practical engagements and commitments of oneself, one's family, even one's community. It can also precipitate efforts to transform not only oneself but also the social and material spaces in which one lives. The moral (or ethical) engine of these efforts of transformation is a "ground project" (as the philosopher Bernard Williams [1981] speaks of it) that I am simply calling "care of the intimate other." I explore the moral complexity of ground projects, practices of care that parents (using the term broadly to include all parenting kin in a family) undertake in circumstances that are fraught and uncertain, when it often seems impossible to find any best good that is worth acting upon, but where, nonetheless, people continue to care about and struggle to obtain some version of a good life. I use the terms *moral* and *ethical* interchangeably throughout. There are theoretical reasons for my doing so, just as – for different theoretical reasons—many scholars differentiate the two. I won't say more at this stage; this is a matter for discussion further down the road. (Especially in chapters 2 and 3.)

The ethnographic heart of this book has emerged from a research project that began in January 1997 and continued until 2011. It has followed African American families residing in Los Angeles County, many from South Central LA. The research has been carried out by a larger, interdisciplinary research team under the direction of Mary Lawlor and myself. I have described the parameters and key questions motivating the research elsewhere (see especially Mattingly 2010b), and I do not go into much detail here. The study is officially over, though a number of us who constituted the core research team continue to be in contact with these families. There have been close to fifty families in the study altogether (and approximately thirty at any one time). Twenty of them participated for more than ten years. Because I have known the families I write about for so many years, I have had the chance to consider, from many angles and over time, what it has meant for various members of the family to undertake these arduous projects of care. Although I rely upon what I have learned from this wide range of participants, in this book I concentrate primarily upon five families. Mostly I speak of mothers or grandmothers, because in our study they have been the ones most involved in bringing up the children (Lawler 2004). However, not only mothers but also fathers, aunts, older siblings, even cousins can play a central role in providing care. Their voices too are periodically heard.

The work of raising "good" children is a "universal function of the family," anthropologists have argued (Ochs and Kremer-Sadlit 2007). Focus upon the family as a primary moral site is especially pertinent within the African American community, where, for many historical, political, and economic reasons, including systematic exclusion from the public life of work and career, the domestic space of the family and the care of children have served as essential ground projects. Many factors, including poverty, have also propelled African American families to be flexible and creative in their kinship arrangements. The importance of family, with a mother or grandmother often functioning as the ethical lynchpin, is a well-known feature of African American life and moral discourse.[1]

In the context of African American families, one cannot overemphasize the centrality of what Collins (2000) has called the "Superstrong Black Mother" as a highly valued moral ideal around which a whole constellation of virtues have been extolled and, in the hands of black feminist scholars, also problematized.[2] This ideal type centers upon the primary task of care for and protecting others, especially one's children.[3] These qualities and virtues include being "self-reliant and resourceful,"[4] "assertive,"[5] "self-sacrificing,"[6] and, above all, as the name implies, "strong." This overarching quality of strength so often associated with the "stereotypical black woman" encompasses a range of other related or synonymous attributes, including being "authoritarian, compelling, competent, courageous, decisive, emphatic, fiery, firm, loud, persistent, powerful, tenacious, vigorous, and zealous" (Blackman 1999:60). Although not all of these characteristics may seem to be virtues, scholars of African American experience have argued their historical necessity from slavery onward and note that they continue to be essential attributes for black women living within a contemporary and still racist America.[7] Strength, in all its many forms, is needed, because the task of caring for and protecting oneself and one's family demands struggle—or to borrow an old expression once used by formerly enslaved black women—it demands one "straggle," which means to "struggle, strive and drag all at once" (Miles 2008:101). Feminists have emphasized that this portrait of good motherhood equates it with a relentless willingness to strive and struggle, even a kind of martyrdom.[8] "Strength" has operated as a "cultural mandate," a moral imperative "to exhibit an automatic endurance to a life perceived as filled with obstacles, unfairness, and tellingly, a lack of assistance from others" (Beauboeuf-Lafontant 2007:31). As a Superstrong Black Woman, one is inevitably guilty, already sentenced. Life itself is a matter of "doing hard time."[9]

Feminists have challenged morally idealized representations of the "Superstrong Black Mother" even when acknowledging that it represents important qualities African American women have had to cultivate. There are resonances between this critical feminist perspective and the views expressed by many of the parents. They would generally concur that being a strong black mother (or father) has meant unrelenting sacrifice and the postponement or abandonment of personal dreams. It has also meant confronting the ways they fall short of this ideal. But I suggest throughout this book that the moral demands these parents face are not adequately captured by the difficulties of living up to the performative requirements of this subject position. It is not merely (though this is no small thing) that they may feel imprisoned by a position that is too difficult to attain, or by the need to perform a role against their own inner feelings or desires. Moral life poses even worse difficulties than this. Performative troubles often pale against the life-and-death struggles so many of their children face and the kind of demands this places upon parents. Again and again, I return to the moral perils parents encounter as they undertake the task of trying to become Superstrong Black Parents. I look especially at how often their lives are threatened by moral tragedy.

The home is obviously a crucial site in which parenting occurs and family life is created, but it is only one of the many moral spaces families traverse in their practices of care. Schools, parks, churches, clinics, neighborhoods—all these are central. Each such social and institutional world is characterized by an array of specific norms and practices. Morally speaking, these are not homogeneous spaces, and they are often conflicting ones. As parents move among them, they encounter and must navigate multiple moral normativities and authorities, including ones that clash with their own sense of a "good life" for their children or for their families. Following families and children into a variety of moral spaces that make distinct and authoritative claims about the "good life" reveals in a particularly vivid way that moral resources for self-making are not contained within particular "local moral worlds" or "regimes of truth" but rather are drawn from an uneasily coexisting "assemblage" of ideals and practices.[10] Moral pluralism characterizes ordinary life. No one ethnography can do justice to all these social spaces, and I have not tried to do so here. I primarily focus on interrelationships among four of them: home, clinic, church, and "street." Although obviously this does not yield a complete picture of the moral repertoire that family members draw upon, it suggests a great deal about its complicated character.

One primary aim of this book is to highlight just how morally complex and uncertain ordinary life can be. It is deeply and confusingly interlaced with matters that seem beyond control and others we might be able to influence. It is a shifting admixture of possibility and necessity. How is it, Marx asked paradoxically, that we make history and also that history makes us? This confusion is of immense *moral* significance to the parents I write about. It has also been of grave concern to moral philosophers, phenomenologists, and, increasingly, anthropologists in the emerging anthropology of morality. (I take this up in greater theoretical detail in the following chapter.)

To think about this feature of everyday life ethnographically, I focus upon events, some large and dramatic, others small and almost invisible. Events, as Jackson has noted, allow us to investigate the "relationship between the forces that act upon us and our capacity for bringing the new into being" (2005: xi). I target events in family life that illustrate with particular clarity the kinds of moral dilemmas and tasks parents face in caring for their children. Each event I describe is in important respects singular and not merely representative of some social category (for example, African American parents with children who have special needs), but the point of dwelling in detail on small moments in small places is not to undertake a tiresome documentation of particularities. Rather, my purpose is to elaborate singular moments precisely in order to speak to moral experiences that have a broad—even existential—significance in illuminating the human plight of caring in the midst of suffering. Attending to singular events allows us to consider how life as lived comprises not only what "actually happened" (what phenomenologists call life's "facticity") but also what *might have happened* as well as what it portends for what *might still happen,* life's possibility.

FIRST PERSON VIRTUE ETHICS

In asking how we can understand the ethical dilemmas and experiences of parents like Tanya, I open an intellectual discussion that is old in philosophy and more recent in anthropology where it is tied to an emerging anthropology of morality. My contribution to this conversation is to outline a first person virtue ethics that draws inspiration from two philosophical quarters, phenomenology and especially the twentieth-century revival of virtue ethics (sometimes called neo-Aristotelian ethics) in moral philosophy. There are a number of key features of this first person ethics that I elaborate throughout the book. Already Tanya's situation, so briefly described, suggests some of them. I begin to sketch these in what follows. My debt to both phenomenology and philosophical virtue ethics will quickly become apparent.

The Good Life

Most centrally, Tanya's situation speaks to her commitment to try to create a good life and what a struggle that can be. It is not only challenging to achieve but difficult to ascertain. No general moral law or rule can address the complexity of her task of discernment because it is utterly embedded within the particularities of her life situation. It is morally demanding because Tanya doesn't just want her son to be physically safe; she wants him to thrive—she wants to create a good and happy life for him. Her concern reflects a basic tenet of virtue ethics. The good life for humans is not merely about surviving but concerns flourishing, Aristotle argued. This notion is sometimes translated as "happiness," but problematically so because it cannot be equated with a mere subjective feeling of pleasure or contentment. Rather, happiness or human flourishing is better understood as something like leading a "life worth living" or a "good life." Moral thriving depends upon the cultivation of wisdom that will allow an agent to discern what is worthy to pursue in her life amid various circumstances.

By foregrounding the importance of moral discernment or judgment, I introduce a deliberative and even reflectively critical component into moral life. Universal rules and calculations cannot replace this activity of discernment. Judgment, in this Aristotelian sense, cannot be reduced to a single choice or an act of will. It is bound up with character and with practices that both express and help in the cultivation of character. But this is not an exercise of judgment or free will on the part of an autonomous moral agent. Virtue ethics inspired by Aristotle is communal. The good life is presumed to be lived in and with community and directed to ideals that encompass collective goods. Intersubjectively held ideals of worthiness are not reducible to mere individual preferences or hedonistic desires.

One of the most significant legacies of the neo-Aristotelian revival is the presumption that human existence concerns process—the "being" of human life is not a set of qualities but rather processes of becoming, that is, its potentiality and its possibilities (Cavell 2004). In ethical terms, cultivating virtue is part of this process of becoming, and it is realized in and through activities. Aristotle regarded *praxis* as directed, most important, to the human cultivation of a good life. This is very much a good life that is *acted*. As such, it is full of frailty and uncertainty, features of everyday life that many neo-Aristotelians have emphasized much more than Aristotle would have likely acknowledged. For classical Greece, "to act in its general sense," Arendt points out, "means to take an initiative, to begin ... to set something into motion" (1958:177). For Aristotle, this beginning was intimately tied to a "sense of an ending" because an action is always tied to a *telos,* "that-for-the-sake-of-which" (Aristotle 1970; Knight 2007:10). But in moral matters, the Aristotelian telos cannot be reduced to a mere goal in the manner of means–ends relationship. Virtuous action is also an end in itself; the process is part of, expresses, so to speak, the telos.

Anthropology has a crucial contribution to make to this ancient philosophical portrayal of human flourishing. It can offer ethnographically grounded depictions of struggles for the good life as contextualized within a variety of different communally shaped ideals of the virtues and the good. An ethnographic focus on how people attempt to realize lives they consider morally worthy, even in the most blighted and unpromising circumstances, has something to contribute to anthropology. It calls attention to the way people consider and evaluate their lives in light of notions of what is ethically good or right. They may fall short, and may be seen by others as falling short, but this does not obviate the presence of such considerations. As Laidlaw puts it: "The claim on which the anthropology of ethics rests is not an evaluative claim that people are good: it is a descriptive claim that they are evaluative" (2014:3; see also Fassin 2008). Such on-going ethical evaluations speak to basic human questions concerning "how we should live and what kind of person we want to be" (Lambek 2008:134). Attention to "the good" or the ethical, understood in this sense, promises to enrich our accounts of action by moving us away from accounts that reduce practical reasoning to an instrumental calculation about how to realize culturally valued ends (Mhyre 1999).

In a provocative essay, Joel Robbins calls for an "anthropology of the good" that has some resonance with earlier anthropological ideals of cultural comparison.[11] The proposal of Robbins and others speaks very closely to the ambitions of this book. Although a focus on the good life and moral striving may seem to promote a naïve unwillingness to recognize the violence that characterizes so much human interaction or the human propensity for evil, this misunderstands what is entailed in such a project. I quote Robbins at some length because of his valuable framing of this enterprise:

> To study the good as anthropologists, we need to be attentive to the way people orientate to and act in a world that outstrips the one most concretely present to them, and . . . avoid dismissing their ideals as unimportant or, worse, as bad-faith alibis for the worlds they actually create. It is not that imaginings of the good cannot be sometimes set aside in practice or put to use in ideological projects that support the continued existence of structures of violence and suffering, but if we assume that ideals always and only get either ignored or deployed in nefarious ways, then the anthropology of the good can never get off the ground. (2013:457)

The point here is not that people are necessarily motivated to be good (rather than, say, malicious or cruel) or that they are never misled by violent or callous ideologies. Rather, the cultural point is that moral striving seems to matter a great deal to people in all sorts of societies. What constitutes the good life may vary widely from society to society, but it is difficult to imagine any community where this does not matter or where, if it has ceased to be important, this does not seem problematic for its members.[12] In fact, what may emerge from a focus on moral striving is not that people manage to live happy and flourishing lives but that they are often plagued by the threat of moral tragedy. The tragic runs through this book as it runs through the lives I write about. How tragedy is created and especially how it is faced—this constitutes one central thread that ties together the stories in the chapters that follow.

The Good Life from a First Person Perspective

What does a first person perspective reveal about moral striving and the good life? Put differently, why is this a first person topic? Tanya's situation again illustrates. Her aspirations for a good life are not something that she simply knows about in a third person sort of way—as moral truths just out there in the world. Rather, they make demands upon her. And, conversely, these commitments and projects give her a "self." The soccer game presents itself to Tanya in a particular kind of way, one informed by her engagements with the world. Her ethical question (Should she let her son play or not?) confronts her not as a universal problem to which an objective normative answer is demanded but rather as an intimately personal one, bound up with her ongoing commitment to her son, her husband, and her efforts to create a good family life—these familial commitments are essential life projects for her. When Williams (1981) speaks of "ground projects," he offers a compelling picture of this mutually constitutive relationship between the self and one's moral projects. Ground projects refer to the kinds of commitments that people find so deep to who they are that they might not care to go on with their lives without them, or would not know themselves if they no longer had them. They include deeply cherished and self-defining ideals, activities, and personal associations.

Put another way, Tanya does not perceive her son's involvement in soccer from a universalizing third person perspective, as one might imagine a health researcher doing. She does not, for example, ponder the statistical probabilities of health and psychological outcomes of children who use wheelchairs playing rough sports. Rather, she asks from "inside," as an engaged actor who finds herself embedded within a particular social and interpersonal situation, a situation in which the results of her actions are deeply consequential for her and those she cares about. Her stance of "care" is a manifestation of something very basic to human experience. To be human is to care about who we are, what we do, what happens to us. Existence just *is* care, Heidegger said. It is this feature of our existence that makes it impossible to adequately characterize humans without adopting a first person starting point. We simply are not the sort of beings who can be summed up by the categories into which we can be placed or the properties we have, in a third person sort of way. Rather, we have a first person orientation to them, we respond to the categories that "name" us and the social practices we participate in. This first person experience is an inextricable aspect of what makes these categories "real." Phenomenology underscores the way that reality presents itself to us as something "out there" only through our own engagement with it.

Phenomenologists have noted that for Aristotle this quality of "given-ness" of experiential phenomena holds true not only for our practical engagements but even for theoretical knowledge. Although theoretical knowledge that humans develop "extend[s] beyond the domain of human concerns," it is grounded in human capabilities for experiencing the world (Baracchi 2008:2). The general point here is that we are not only embedded in social practices that existed before we came along, we respond to those practices through a stance of commitment—they matter to us, they speak to us and make demands on us. It is this mattering, or things being "at stake" as Kleinman (2006) has often put it, that gives them their first person character. (Notably, such a stance can include a range of responses, including being alienated from projects in which we find ourselves embedded.)

Acknowledging our responsivity vis-à-vis the world, or put differently, the way that the world and our response to it are inextricably entangled, challenges third person accounts of persons (Wentzer 2014). We are, as Charles Taylor has said, "self-interpreting animals." This claim presupposes a certain understanding of what it means to have a self at all. A self is "identified with the very first personal givenness of the experiential phenomena. . . . To be conscious of oneself, consequently, is not to capture a pure self that exists in separation from the stream of consciousness, but rather entails just being conscious of an experience in its first personal mode of givenness; it is a question of having first personal access to one's own experiential life" (Zahavi 2005:106). This is not to suggest that our experiences are in any simple sense clearly available to us or give us an unquestioned understanding of what presents itself. It is a commonplace truth that we may wonder if what our senses have told us is, in fact, the case. What's more, Lear comments, we have what he calls an "ethical fantasy life," an "inchoate sense that there is a remainder to life, something that is not captured in life as it is so far experienced" (2000:163, cited in Lambek 2008:142).

This experiential givenness, in all its shadowy complexity, can be contrasted with a "third person perspective" that begins with categories themselves. These serve as the primary unit of analysis and provide the focal point for explanatory attention. In Heidegger's phenomenology, third person ontologies are explicitly contested. Within third person positions, Wentzer (articulating Heidegger's challenge) states, "Things ontologically classified by categorical distinctions are what they are according to their essence or species, or rather, according to their purposefulness and function in practical dealings . . ." (Wentzer 2012:311). But this mode of characterization is not sufficient for humans because it violates our own basic human self-experience. We do not experience ourselves, ontologically, merely as a type of being, a member of a species. We are not simply determined by these categories, properties, and practices but also in orienting to them and experiencing our lives in light of them, we are capable of putting them into question.[13]

It becomes clear that whatever a first person perspective might mean, it extends far beyond a term designating some individual person's inner life of experience. In fact, what is challenged is this very split between subjective and objective.[14] The phenomenological tradition involves the strong claim that objectivity itself is but one attitude within the range of necessarily engaged and first person ways in which we are enmeshed with the world. Michael Jackson (2005) speaks of this enmeshment as a kind of fusion, referring not only to our social relationships with others but also to the physical environments we inhabit, stressing the active, embodied nature of this engagement. Objective or third person descriptions merely offer one way to represent the world—and ourselves. They suggest one interpretive possibility, a possibility that may have its uses but can also be misleading. Subjectivity, in this extended and philosophical sense, is necessarily the name for our primary relationship to anything "out there," including the ways that reality is apprehended and named by us in the manner of the objective, external world, a world of facts and impersonal objects.

Moral Becoming as Experiment: Moral Laboratories

I suggest what at first take may seem a surprising trope for illuminating a first person ethics by considering social spaces as potential moral laboratories. Tanya's situation also illustrates that moral efforts at discerning a momentary best good are not simply matters of personal introspection and reflection. They are—very often—moments of action that call for the transformation of social and physical spaces. Soccer is not the same game with a wheelchair and a medically fragile child as part of it; the field, the rules of the sport, all of these are subtly reinvented by the players in accommodation of this nonstandard scene of action. Parks, clinic waiting rooms, soccer fields, as we will see, all can become the unlikely grounds for moral experimentation and the creation of transformative experiences. These emergent and fleeting moral laboratories provide vantage points on familiar or prior ways of seeing, acting, believing that are actively brought into question. They are also experiments in hope and possibility. They suggest possible futures even while taking place in some all-too-real, and often quite ordinary, present. The actions themselves may seem mundane enough, but they may also function in this experimental way, as actions within possible narratives of transformation, moments in possible lives.

I have chosen this trope of the laboratory precisely to emphasize that these are spaces of possibility, ones that create experiences that are also experiments in how life might or should be lived. Each experiment holds its perils. Each provokes moments of critique, especially self-critique. These are not obvious laboratories; nor are they obvious spaces for moral reflection, moral practice, and moral deliberation. And yet, each serves in this way. It took me a long time to notice the way such spaces were created by families, by children, sometimes by clinicians as well. It is not always apparent that anything of significance is going on, or that there is a kind of moral crisis or dilemma that is being addressed, especially in children's playful moments. I have come to notice the weight of such spaces only over a long acquaintance with the people I write about here.

Although throughout this book I frequently consider moral laboratories and moral reflections as related to clinical diagnoses, medical problems, and health care, any clinical window into the suffering of these families reveals little about their moral dilemmas or hopes. Hope as dependent upon the dream of a clinical cure or rescue is perhaps not beside the point, but it is certainly a small part of the point. I had no idea when the study began that I would find myself in geographical—not to mention imaginative and moral—spaces that were such a distance from the way that medical problems were framed by health professionals. Nor did I realize, when our study began, how caught up I would become in the family and in parental hopes and dilemmas that might seem irrelevant to anything medical but were, in fact, of the essence in shaping how children—even those with severe disabilities—fared.

At first glance, a laboratory does not seem a very auspicious metaphor to handle this first person portrait of moral becoming. After all, the lab is a quintessential scene of modernity and postmodernity, a cultural imaginary that includes not only lab rats, test tubes, and white-coated scientists, but also the "onco-mouse," the "ibf stem cell," and all sorts of other dazzling and unprecedented creatures. It has often served as both trope and exemplar for systems frameworks (like Actor Network Theory) that emphasize the interrelatedness of human and nonhuman actors (such as computers) in producing effects in the world. This is a very far cry from first person framework I propose. The laboratory I have in mind, a *moral laboratory,* is a different kind of imaginative space. It is a metaphorical realm in which experiments are conducted in all kinds of places and where participants are neither mere objects of study nor entities in some cyborgic system but rather researchers or experimenters of their own lives.

This is a scene of action in which the "new" is inaugurated, where new experiences are created. Notably, one of the primary definitions of experience is "experiment" *(Oxford English Dictionary);* it is this relationship between experience and experiment, the experimental nature of experience itself, that the laboratory trope highlights. In this moral laboratory, participants are not only working with the odds but also, in important ways, *against* them. The possible is pitted against the predictable. This is a laboratory of unique human actions, a space for the production of beginnings, which turn out to be miracles of a sort. We can get a sense of this moral scene in Arendt's description of the inaugural moment when an "I," a moral self, emerges. With action, she argues, humans are able to create something new—to begin something unexpected. And in this creation of "the new" they create themselves. "The new always happens against the overwhelming odds of statistical laws and their probability which for all practical, everyday purposes amounts to certainty," she writes. "And the new therefore always appears in the guise of a miracle" (1958:178).

Moral laboratories that produce the possible (as against the probable), that produce, in other words, singular acts that transform material and social space and create moral selves, are marked with a radical uncertainty. We might be able to begin something—against the odds—something new. A soccer game reinvented so that a boy using a wheelchair can play--this, in my view, exemplifies just such a "miracle," a small moment of natality. Soccer is "reborn," albeit locally. But this rebirth holds no guarantees; it offers no predicable future and it brings with it unanticipated risks. As Arendt tells us, any "miracle" and the "rebirth" it provides the doer is precarious from the start. We have little control of where that beginning will go, what the consequences of our initial actions will be, and we must, as we say, "suffer the consequences." "Because the actor always moves among and in relation to other acting beings," Arendt remarks, "he is never merely a 'doer' but always and at the same time a sufferer. To do and to suffer are like opposite sides of the same coin . . ." (1958:190).

Considering a soccer game as a kind of moral laboratory illuminates how Tanya becomes (reluctantly) willing to experiment with her own ideas of the limits of her son's capabilities and the capabilities of the children and parents around him. This game creates an event that transforms her view of her son and herself. Tanya's dilemma over the soccer game reveals the intricacy of what goes into making a moral judgment within any particular situation—and its vulnerability as well. In the name of one kind of "good" (keeping her child physically safe—no small feat with Andy), she resists her husband's attempts to let him play this rough sport. She judges a very different best good than her husband in this context. But she recognizes that in doing so, she must give up another best good, which is allowing her son to do something highly valued by his father, something that father and son try to share in many different ways (as when Andy "shot hoops" as a younger child).

Tanya deeply appreciates her husband's great involvement in raising their son and his pride in doing so. And yet, in this case, she discerns it too dangerous. She is by no means the master of this social space of soccer; her judgment about the best good depends upon her reading of fellow participants in the game. What can she ask and expect not only of children playing on the field but also of their parents? How far will people be willing to accommodate a boy using a wheelchair? How much ingenuity and compassion can she expect from others? Ultimately, for Tanya, the soccer field becomes a space of hope—of opportunities she had not dreamed possible. It also becomes a space of critique—a reflective examination of her own assumptions and what she could ask of her son, of herself, of the community around her. A soccer field is hardly an obvious space of social experiment, moral critique, or personal transformation. And yet, it emerges as a kind of moral laboratory that is created in the midst of everyday life.

Narrativity and the Temporality of Ethics

Experiences generated in moral laboratories are transformative not only (or even especially) in and of themselves but because they serve as experiments in unfolding lives, giving them a temporal depth that is so integral to any analysis of moral becoming. Tanya's problem of the soccer game is posed to her *in time*; it belongs to history of commitments and memories but also is anticipatory, intimating hopes and aspirations that travel backward and forward in time, shaping the way any particular moment or event is experienced. Even the past becomes different as the present and future change shape. This is a feature of human experience that phenomenologists refer to as "historicity." What they mean by this is not simply that any particular event (say, a soccer game) or person (say, Tanya) has a history or is born into history. Rather, they are saying something about the temporal features of experience itself as it is humanly lived.

The "present" is not experienced as an isolated incident. Nor is it experienced as a next event emerging in linear fashion from a past. Rather, the phenomenological claim is that what presents itself to someone for experience is always situated within a temporal arc that encompasses past experiences and prefigures future ones: human time evinces a "three fold present."[15] The scene from the soccer game I initially described was a moment lived by Tanya and her family in a temporal horizon that included not only their individual and familial pasts but also possible futures that were foreshadowed but uncertain. Both past and future potential experiences shape the perceptions and meanings of any particular soccer game.

This phenomenal complexity of time is integral to the conception of a first person self. Aristotle's practical philosophy depends upon some notion of a self that continues through time.[16] Even perception requires the analytic primacy of an individual who has some temporal coherence and continuity, phenomenologists have contended, an individual who experiences over time, as Aristotle also believed.[17] But the Aristotelian presumption of an enduring self has been particularly attractive to Anglo-American moral philosophers reviving virtue ethics. Aristotelian ethics cannot do without a very robust notion of the arc of a life and some kind of biographical integrity. The whole notion of cultivating one's character depends upon it. An individual agent is a historical being, one who endures over time and is imbued with a complex internal life. This is a "thick" self (that is, socially embedded, historically singular, enduring, and emotionally complex) rather than a "thin" or "fractured" one. So, for example, in introducing his notion of "ground projects" Williams calls upon "the basic importance for our thought of the ordinary idea of a self or person which undergoes changes of character, as opposed to an approach which, even if only metaphorically, would dissolve the person, under changes of character, into a series of 'selves'" (1981:5). Such a self is analytically demanded if ethics is concerned with "the cultivation of character, the training of moral emotions, the centrality of intention, motive and the inner life" and if it is directed not merely to "isolated acts of choice, but also, and more importantly, on the whole course of an agent's moral life, its patterns of commitment, conduct, and also passion" (Hursthouse 1999:170).

There is a temporality to our projects of care that leads many scholars (and I am one of them) to insist that there is an inherent narrativity to ethical practice and its self-constituting nature. Commitments and projects have a history, and, in taking them up or responding to them, we become part of a history. Cultivating virtues as part of these commitments and projects belongs to a task of moral becoming, and this, too, implies the narrativity of moral life. It presumes a self that has a strongly marked narrative character. Both phenomenologists and virtue ethicists have elaborated this feature of human temporality in narrative terms; lived time unfolds for us in a plot-like way. A present experience is a kind of middle that emerges from beginnings that continue to be revised and endings that are foreshadowed and prefigured but remain in suspense.

This is in some ways analogous to our experience of reading or hearing a story, a common philosophical parallel. We anticipate what will happen next not only based upon the events that have already happened but upon our sense of the unfolding "whole" of which each story event is a part. This sense of the whole (the "plot") unfolds temporally in our experience of reading or hearing a story—not only future anticipated events but also past events are revised in our imagination in this process.[18] But the analogy between reading a story and living a life takes us only so far because it tends to disguise both the agentive and the moral aspects of lived experience. In "real-life" situations, especially ones that present us with dilemmas that have a certain urgency, this temporal complexity manifests itself to us not only as readers of our lives but as doers of them. We are called to respond. And our response has a history, becomes part of a history.[19]

The trope of the quest or journey is often invoked by moral philosophers, suggesting a familiar, ancient, and culturally widespread narrative framing of lived experience as a path of moral becoming, one that has been given special attention within philosophical virtue ethics. It gains narrative specificity as instantiated in American, and more specifically African American, family life. The overarching dramatic narrative of the perilous quest is variously emplotted by the families I write about as heroic battle, domestic comedy, moral tragedy, elegy, and spiritual pilgrimage. These narrative strains, or plotlines, are not mutually exclusive but are lived out and furthered simultaneously. Even plots with a cosmic narrative reach are also deeply domesticated in household routines, squabbles, jokes, and rituals. Such a narrative framing might seem to presume an overly coherent self, a life unfurling with orderly precision. But I suggest something very different: that narrative provides a useful approach for investigating projects of moral becoming riddled by uncertain possibilities and informed by pluralistic moral values, concerns, and communities.

For Tanya, the whole soccer quandary—developing over several years as she and her husband initially debate it and then continuing as soccer games are played and she watches worriedly from the sidelines—is both a difficulty in its own right ("an event," so to speak) and part of a larger unfolding life. It is eventful as an episode in her moral project of becoming a "good mother." But goodness is not a straightforward cumulative achievement. The point here, speaking again phenomenologically, is that being a "good mother" is not a static matter. It does not mean merely inhabiting a fixed category and doing the things that this role normatively prescribes. Cultural norms of "good mothering" can serve as guidelines, but they do not pre-decide for Tanya what good mothering should look like in the variety of circumstances life presents to her.

The vocabulary of moral becoming also speaks to the outcomes of Tanya's decisions here. She comes to experience these soccer games as life changing, fundamentally reorienting her understanding of what good mothering (for her at least) entails. Soccer playing prompts a generative shift in her own moral understanding of her project of care. Put narratively, these soccer games instigate a reimagining of the kind of moral story she is in. I speak of this process as a task of *narrative re-envisioning,* a further elaboration of what I have elsewhere called a "narrative phenomenology" of social practice (Mattingly 2010b). By narrative re-envisioning, I mean the activity of coming to see oneself in a new way, coming to reform one's sense of possibility and reframe one's commitments. But it also includes the task of becoming a kind of person capable of formulating and acting upon commitments that one deems ethical. The idea that one lives a life that is, in some way, one's own, and that is a moral project, is an indispensable intuition for the parents and families I describe. This narrative work speaks most directly to the moral and not merely to the competent aspect of practical action. Narrative re-envisioning is also very embodied, occurring in and through participation in social worlds.

Narrative re-envisioning extends beyond personal life trajectories and the ground projects that configure them meaningfully. Life trajectories are embedded within larger social and historical horizons that are crucial in shaping personal commitments. MacIntyre contends that what is "at stake" in any particular act is necessarily connected to a narrative picture of the self. This is not an explicitly told story but an interpretive framework that agents draw upon in assessing what actions they ought to take. Actions, especially ones that involve clearly moral assessments, are not undertaken and cannot even be interpreted by others without some interpretation of "longer and longest-term intentions . . . and how the shorter-term intentions are related to the longer." Longer-term intentions speak to a person's sense of self, MacIntyre suggests. In discerning what a person is up to in light of what is at stake, for them, we are referring to their longer-term intentions, which means, as he puts it, "we are involved in writing a narrative history" (1981:193).

Following a somewhat different but complementary line of argument, Charles Taylor puts narrative at the center of moral action by exploring what it is that gives us a self in the first place. He asserts that it is primarily through having things "at stake" that one has a self at all: "We are selves only in that certain issues matter for us. What I am as a self, my identity, is essentially defined by the way things have significance for me. . . . We are only selves insofar as we move in a certain space of questions, as we seek and find an orientation to the good" (1989:34). It is impossible to speak of understanding a person, Taylor continues, "in abstraction from his or her self-interpretations," and these self-interpretations concern what is of significance (1989:34).

Taylor is particularly eloquent in arguing for a narrative framework that encompasses both the narrative features of a self and also of action. What is moral for us, he argues, speaks to our sense of what is significant, and "significance" is necessarily a moral term because it calls upon this "orientation to the good" (1989:34). The moral is only understandable, he further argues, in terms of "what is of crucial importance to us." But, in a kind of circularity he insists on the interweaving of self-understanding, character, and action. Our actions and what is of significance are self-defining features of who we are. He states, "To know who I am is a species of knowing where I stand. My identity is defined by the commitments and identifications which provide the frame or horizon within which I can try to determine from case to case what is good, or valuable, or what ought to be done, or what I endorse or oppose. In other words, it is the horizon within which I am capable of taking a stand" (1989:27).

In a manner that echoes Williams's concept of a ground project, Taylor tells us this framework is so important that if people were without it, they would be "at sea"—they would lose their way in "moral space" (1989:29). Taylor further insists that this orientation makes sense only in light of a narratively understood self: "This sense of the good has to be woven into my understanding of my life as an unfolding story."[20] Our self-identity is first and foremost built around morality—orientations to "the good." Iris Murdoch calls us "moral pilgrims," a conceit that speaks to the questlike narrative structure of this moral self that is always in the process of becoming.[21] This narrative sense of self is not an "optional extra," Taylor argues. Drawing on Heidegger's construal of the temporal structure of being, he states, "In order to have a sense of who we are, we have to have a notion of how we have become, and of where we are going" (1989:47). We cannot operate without this minimal narrative understanding of our lives.

The robust first person perspective offered here ties who I am to those matters that "have significance for me" (Taylor 1989:34; Williams 1981). But this "me" is historical and social before it is individual. It begins with my induction into a community, or set of communities. As Taylor puts it, "One cannot be a self on one's own." A self is always constructed by reference to some defining communities. This dialogical self depends upon what Taylor calls "'webs of interlocution'" (1989:36). After I have been raised in such communities, I may "innovate"—that is, "develop an original way of understanding myself and human life . . . which is in sharp disagreement with my family and background" (1989:35). But even here, our communities are not left behind. They provide our spaces of conversation. Taylor is trying to create a picture of the moral self that avoids two common notions that are both problematic. He contrasts this dialogical view of how moral selves are created from *both* individualist understandings of the moral self *and* a social constructionism that views selves as pre-given by public convention.

Here again, Tanya's situation serves as useful illustration of this social narrativity of projects of self-transformation. For Tanya, soccer stands as a moment that generates a new willingness to battle for her son. It is another moment that confronts her with a demand that she cultivate virtues that will aid in care of her son. One virtue—one might call it courage—is key to her own sense of her transformative journey. Tanya, like many parents in this study, told stories about the misery of learning that compliance to clinical authorities is not the answer to good care or a good life. Tanya learned to demand better investigative care for her child from her own mother. Tanya's mother was a nurse. (I quote here from a passage in the *Paradox of Hope*.)

A few months after Tanya's first child was born, her mother suspected that he was not developing properly. She became furious that Tanya's pediatrician (who was near retirement) was missing obvious cues of serious cognitive delay. She tried to get Tanya to confront him. Tanya did not want to. Her mother asked her: "Who is this old man? Is he asking you this? Is he asking you that?" When her mother confronted her, she "would get upset with her." She remembers their arguments. "They know what they're doing," she would tell her mother. "Stop it, stop it, stop it!" But her mother persisted and finally, when her son was four months old, they went to see the pediatrician together. This is how Tanya described their encounter:

> He said [to her mother], "Oh granny, he's a preemie and this is something they go through." He was just like, "Oh, they take longer to do things, and you just gotta relax." And she says, "Listen, I'm a nurse and I've dealt with people like you. Sometimes you gotta just pay attention to the signs. And I don't know if you're stupid or if you're smart, but I know one thing. You're going to pay attention to this baby because I'm going to find the best lawyer that I can find or take my daughter out of this pediatrician's office." And I'm sitting there in shock that she's talking to him this way. And then he calmed down and said, "I'm sorry, I apologize. You're right. We'll insist that he goes to a specialist and make sure there's no harm, because he's not tracking. You're right."

The pediatrician finally made referrals to specialists. And this is how Tanya ended up getting a diagnosis of cerebral palsy for her son. (Mattingly 2010b:61–62)

When Tanya's mother confronts her physician, who finally refers her four-month-old infant to a specialist and she discovers he has cerebral palsy, this is not merely a clinical matter. Tanya tells her story as part of a narration of how she had to become transformed herself to be a good mother to her severely disabled child. She must "find strength" not just to bear the difficulties of raising a medically fragile child but also to learn how to battle physicians when necessary.

Tanya has fought many battles over the years not only for her child but also for other children with special needs. She lives in South Central Los Angeles, a low-income community where services are notoriously inadequate. Through a great deal of strategic maneuvering, she was able to move her son into an elite magnet school in the Los Angeles suburbs where she joined a group of wealthy parents developing a new special education program. But this did not solve her problem as she had hoped. Despite the resources of this rich, predominantly white community, she still could not get her son the kind of education she believed he deserved. "School," she says with a sigh. "I'm so disillusioned by it all." When she "drops in on occasion" to see what is going on in her son's classroom, what she sees is "day care." "The special ed. kids sit in the room and look at the walls," she complains. "You're like, where's the curriculum? Where's the structure for these kids?"

Despite all of her efforts and efforts of other parents, she has been in continual and discouraging strife with the principal and other teachers of regular education classes.

> We fight ten times over in this school to make ourselves noticed that we want to be a part [of the school]. We're parents that contribute and do what we can, but we're not regarded or respected. Only when they need to show, "Oh we have that handicap room over there. Can you give us a grant? Because we're really a great school." But when making us a part of it, they don't want to regard us since that might make some people feel uncomfortable. There's been certain teachers sayin' "We don't want the kindergarteners [with them]. They might scare the kindergarteners. We don't want them to go with us on field trips or go to the auditorium and stuff." And I just—I don't know. I can't get mad. It's like how many times can you cry? How many times can you get mad? But what can you do?

The ethical here is intimately intertwined with the political, a point presumed by Aristotle that continues to be emphasized by many moral philosophers and anthropologists.[22] By noting this connection, I mean to emphasize the importance of the community, including the civic sphere, as intertwined with personal and familial projects of care. While this may include, as it increasingly does for Tanya, an advocacy role that challenges institutional structures in the name of justice, this need not be the case. It would be far too restrictive to equate the concept of moral agency with political activism. For Tanya, however, her commitments have brought her into increasingly public arenas. Her journey has meant re-envisioning her own subject position in an explicitly political way even as she has become exhausted by the futility of many of her efforts: "I'm just tired. I'm tired of being an adversary of the school system. I'm ready to sit in front of these congressmen and say, you know, 'Walk a year in my shoes and then sit there and tell me that you can make laws like this.'" A confrontation she has taken on with special vehemence concerns inclusion rights for children with special needs. What has been especially frustrating is that she has also tried to help the school as a whole, believing that by doing so the administration would, as they had promised, include the special needs children in schoolwide activities like field trips or allow them out on the playground with others. "We were promised inclusion. I was a mom fighting. I was working my butt off, volunteering, doing fundraisers, being a part of the silent auction."

Tanya situates herself within a much broader historical narrative of populist social justice movements, the black civil rights movement in particular. She is not alone in this; many parents in our study linked their battles with clinicians, school districts, and the like to civil rights. However, she has been especially explicit in seeing her efforts not only as a personal battle but as part of a needed "revolution." She remarked once, her voice passionate with resolve: "It's what started things like the Civil Rights movement. It's what started things like, I don't know (she gives a small laugh) how revolutions start. This has got to stop. This attitude that these kids can't learn (she hits the table for emphasis) or these kids can't be treated with respect or regard." She may laugh self-consciously when she suggests that her efforts could help start a "revolution," but her ongoing efforts show how serious she is.

We can see in her word how intertwined the experience of suffering is with strivings and imaginings for a good life at a collective level. Although the kind of moral efforts I describe here have a distinctively American cast and are rooted in an African American history, they speak to a phenomenon common in a wide range of societies where suffering itself can serve as a cultural resource for moral striving and growth. So, for example, the Yapese, as described by Throop (2010b), make an important distinction between "mere suffering"—pain that happens to an individual that seems to have no moral purpose—and "suffering for," a highly valued cultural virtue in which one learns to endure pain with patience and stoicism because it is connected to one's contributions to the greater good of one's community.

Tanya's trajectory of moral becoming and social transformation might sound like a story of moral progress. Sometimes Tanya sees it this way. But its tragic dimensions are here too. Again and again she has revealed how her re-envisioned commitments and the concomitant political enlargement of her ground project of care have created new moral vulnerabilities. She is always exhausted and often defeated. She wonders if she has sacrificed too much, putting her family life in jeopardy by the political commitments she has taken up with such fervor.

The Everyday and Its Subversive Resources: Critiquing the Morally Normative

I have begun to suggest a portrait of moral transformation and the moral striving surrounding it that is at once experimental, even perilous, traversing private and public life while also deeply embedded in the routines of everyday care. Although many anthropologists have sought to distinguish ordinary action and its norm-governed morality from something that could properly be called a deliberative ethical moment,[23] this is not the direction that I take. Instead, I foreground the ordinary as a prime site of moral work.[24] The type of transformation I describe is not something that occurs *apart* from everyday action in a moment of moral crisis but is accomplished in the midst of the everyday as the normative becomes subject to experiment and problematization. I link experiment and narrative re-envisioning to moral transformation in a specific sense. Obviously, on the one hand, transformation is inevitable in our lives. Our biology dictates this. So, too, does our social community. We are reassigned subject positions based upon our passages through life, upon our changing ages, our marriages, our children, our physical declines, and the like. On the other hand, the very act of carrying out ground projects (like caring for one's children) may involve the transformation of understandings of these projects and positions, conscious effortful tasks of moral becoming that involve experiments in social and material spaces as well as personal selves. It is transformation of this latter sort that I have in mind.

I suggest that the moral ordinary can be more morally subversive than many scholars have presumed. I believe it is important to explore the moral ordinary as a resource for critique and transformation as connected to a "we" and an "I." Perhaps, too, there are resources that everyday persons sometimes draw upon to discover contingency in what seemed necessary or to experiment with moral possibilities that transgress or expand their moral universes. So, too, the contingencies of the ordinary can present resources for moral creativity and experimentation. I pay particular attention to the workings of an indigenous hermeneutics of critique even for those who must live with so few resources and so little social capital.

Throughout the book, I consider several primary resources for transformation and critique. These speak both to the first person efforts of an "I" and a "we" but also to the cultural resources and conditions that they draw upon. The following are taken up and explored: (1) the capacity of people to introduce scenic violations in social spaces that experiment with the social and moral ordinary; (2) the way projects of moral becoming may encourage people to create multiple and even rival future selves; (3) the first person capability of taking a third person perspective on oneself in order to subject third person categories and norms to evaluation and critique; (4) the way that moral norms can generate incommensurable goods that produce situations of moral tragedy and demand a critique of those norms; (5) the presence of multiple and even rival moral schemes within a social community; (6) the resources even within what might seem like hegemonic practices and discourse for critique, modification, and sometimes subversion.

Introducing a first person account of moral becoming within the domains of everyday life provides a way to focus on the structural conditions that produce morality as lived experience. It also offers an avenue for considering the cultural categories and moral norms that so powerfully shape it. If one avoids both structural determinism and a dualistic account of moral life that pitches an unreflective everyday existence against the rare transgressive or deliberative ethical moment, one can begin to uncover how the cultural provides vehicles for reflection, critique, and transformation—even, perhaps, revolution. To recognize the mysteries of the everyday one must look with detailed care at how social conditions become dialectical for people living with them. It takes a close gaze to notice the way small experiments undertaken to address various moral troubles can sometimes spark critiques of the normative as well as efforts to transform the conditions of existence. Tragedy becomes visible too, even as life's possibilities are exposed. Hope and despair, moral aspiration and moral failure—these are close travel companions.

I have chosen this trope of the laboratory to emphasize that as part of the moral work African American parents undertake, everyday spaces can become spaces of possibility, ones that create experiences that are also experiments in how life might or should be lived. Each experiment holds its perils. Each provokes moments of critique, especially self-critique, but also sometimes challenge of the social and moral categories in which it is placed. This includes not only stigmatized categories but also highly idealized ones like the "Superstrong Black Mother." Looking at the experimental features of everyday moral life or efforts at transformation does not yield an optimistic picture. But it does allow us to take a dialectical and even paradoxical formulation of ethical and political life seriously. I focus on "making history" (with a small *h*) projects that arise not because people have some grand ambitions to change the world or a political cheeriness about their capabilities but because of what they often perceive as an unwanted necessity—propelled by the sheer suffering and moral trouble that arises in their tasks to care for their children they find themselves in projects of moral and political transformation.

A PHILOSOPHICAL ANTHROPOLOGY
OF MORAL POSSIBILITY

In his fascinating book, *Radical Hope,* the philosopher Jonathan Lear defines philosophical anthropology in a manner that holds promise for anthropology. He considers an anthropologically informed case concerning Plenty Coups, the "last great chief of the Crow nation" (2006:1). Following the physical and cultural devastation after the buffalo disappeared and the Crow were confined to a reservation, Plenty Coups declares to the white man interviewing him that there are no more stories to tell. After this time, Plenty Coups states, "Nothing happened" to the Crow. Lear ponders this puzzling statement: How can it be that "nothing happened" when the Crow continued to exist? Lear puzzles in a manner he believes quite different from the way anthropologists would. As he puts it, "Unlike an anthropological study, I am not primarily concerned with what *actually happened* to the Crow tribe or any other tribe. I am concerned rather with the *field of possibilities* in which all human endeavors gain meaning . . ." (2006:7, italics added). He elaborates further. "A philosophical inquiry may rely on historical and anthropological accounts . . . but ultimately it wants to know not about actuality but about possibility" (2006:9). He ties this investigation to the problem of ethics—the question of how we ought to live within certain possible circumstances.

Without detracting from the considerable resources philosophy brings to this question, I suggest that anthropologists work on the problem not only of actualities but also of possibilities and their ethical implications. Furthermore—and this is one of Lear's most important points—this is not a question for academics alone. It is also one posed by people—or we might better say posed *to* people—by the circumstances of their lives. The reason this is a concern for anthropologists is because "actuality" consists not simply of things that happen but also of things that might happen (in phenomenological terms, anticipatory or prospective experience) as well as things that might have happened—a history not only of facts but also of past possibilities and roads not taken.

Put in terms of morality, a philosophical task for anthropologists is to consider how cultural conditions pose not only conditions of normative actuality—guiding what can "actually happen"—but also conditions of possibility governing what might happen. Carrithers suggests that perhaps anthropological knowledge is "not a knowledge of struc-

tures alone but also of spacious possibilities and of unintended consequences that crowd closely around certainty" (2005:434). To investigate
these "spacious possibilities" that "crowd closely around certainty," we
might ask, What are the subjunctive potentialities available in certain
cultural and structural circumstances? How do culturally normative
practices not only reproduce themselves but also contain within them
resources for their own challenge? How might they provide provocations for what Arendt calls "natality"—moral striving in which people
try to bring something new (even statistically improbable) into being?
How is this potentiality bound up with suffering, even moral tragedy?
Although Lear—and many anthropologists—consider this under situations of extraordinary moral threat or crisis, I continue to ponder such
questions in light of a perilous moral ordinary.

WHAT FOLLOWS

The book divides into three parts. Part I ("First Person Virtue Ethics")
includes this chapter and the following one. These provide the overall
framing argument. Part II ("Moral Becoming and the Everyday")
includes chapters 3 through 6. It is especially focused on how character
is cultivated as part of on-going experiments in everyday life. Part III
("Moral Pluralism as Cultural Possibility") consists of chapters 7
through 9. It most directly tackles the cultural and political dimensions
of my argument. Chapters 7 and 8, in particular, consider intersections
between the different moral terrains people traverse, looking at conflicting moralities as resources for cultural critique and attempts at social
transformation.

In Chapter 1, I have begun to outline the primary claims concerning a
first person virtue ethics that I continue to develop throughout the book.
Chapter 2 further elaborates what is entailed in a first person version of
virtue ethics in an explicitly debating style. I argue that it is important to
look at the contrasts between a first person virtue ethics and a third person discursive one inspired especially by Foucault. I examine ways that
these positions challenge rather than support one another despite their
many areas of overlap. I particularly highlight conceptual divides regarding the status of the "self." Although I pay special attention to anthropological voices, the question raised—why we need a first person version of
virtue ethics—speaks to a much broader interdisciplinary conversation.
This chapter goes into considerable detail about these two traditions and
will be of far greater interest to some readers than to others.

Chapters 3 and 4 center upon family life. I explore everyday routines as home experiments, introducing an extended household presided over by Delores (the grandmother matriarch) but also by two of her adult daughters, Marcy and Sasha, and their six children. Following this family through several key events, I ask what is at stake, conceptually, in speaking of the "everyday" and locate ethics within the ordinary. These chapters explore how routines are revised or invented in response to the changing circumstances of the family's life. Chapter 4 documents how a household accident challenges the harmony of the family. In response to this accident, Sasha undergoes an arduous project of becoming a new kind of mother and trying to inhabit a new kind of family. I elaborate the notion of narrative re-envisioning introduced in the first chapter and examine it as a form of social and dialogical reflection and action. As part of this, Sasha experiments with new ways for her son to inhabit the household. These experiments are challenged by Delores, who initiates others. As compared to the kind of experimentation I write about in other chapters, these experiments are very small scale and may appear inconsequential. However, when embedded within the context of the family journey and its efforts to repair the moral damage that the accident caused, the experimental qualities of the most quotidian practices become visible.

Chapter 5 opens with an ordinary clinical scene of a child with a severe chronic illness. It involves an ongoing debate between a mother and clinicians, especially her daughter's primary physician, a hematologist who is treating her daughter for sickle cell anemia. This mother, clinically informed and passionately involved in her child's care, strenuously advocates for a highly risky and experimental bone marrow transplant procedure that the hematologist deems far too medically unsafe. Why is the mother so ready to pursue something so dangerous? What is at stake for her, morally speaking? I explore how her day-to-day challenges of cultivating the maternal virtues necessary to fulfill one best good for her daughter place her in a situation of moral incommensurability. She finds herself inextricably caught in a moral tragedy.

Chapter 6 focuses on the experimental nature of action in a way that provides a place to retheorize the relationship between narrative and self-becoming. I suggest that rather than considering the self as both linear and coherent, it is better considered as subjunctive. We are selves "in suspense" (Mattingly 2009, 2010a). I consider the situation of Andrena and her daughter Belinda, who is critically ill with cancer. The problem for Andrena is not merely that her four-year-old girl may die (as clinicians predict likely) but that Andrena will either lose hope while her daughter is still alive or, if her daughter dies, she will be so grief stricken that she will not be able to go on living. This chapter, more than any of the others, shows how moral experimentation can happen in all kinds of places. Such events as a visit to a neighboring mother, a birthday party at Chuck E. Cheese, a visit to a new school—all these moments and spaces are mobilized in a kind of "what if?" experiment in which Andrena actively cultivates two incommensurable future stories at the same time—one where her daughter dies, one where she lives. This experimental stance allows her to practice the virtues of a mother who does not give up hope for her child while also cultivating the strength that will be needed if she must bear the pain of her daughter's death. Her efforts not only concern her ability to care for her child in what she deems the "best good" way, but also to try to care for her future self, to guard against the temptation of suicide.

Chapter 7 asks the primary question that motivates chapters 7 and 8: How can the moral ordinary provide a place to critique and contest it? This chapter takes us into a neonatal intensive care unit (NICU) where parents watch over their critically ill newborn. I look at the NICU as a moral laboratory and a setting for multiple and competing moral imaginaries. In the situation I examine, the parents are locked in a battle with clinicians over the experimental procedures they ask to be carried out on behalf of their baby. This is a familiar battle—the topic of many a medical ethics case. However, it gains moral depth when these clinical experiments are embedded within the parents' attempts to transform their family and themselves, to cultivate the kinds of virtues that make them good parents to all their children. This chapter also investigates how one authoritative moral discourse (a spiritual one) is pitted against another (a biomedical one).

In chapter 8, I return yet again to Delores's extended household. Here, many competing moral spaces and discourses are brought to bear upon one another: the street, the church, and the home. When one of Delores's grandchildren is murdered outside his house, this sparks conversations by family members and others, both on the street and in the church at the funeral, about who is responsible for his death and what kinds of moral transformation his death seems to demand. Here, moral laboratories also become political laboratories where authoritative moral discourses and practices are directly critiqued and challenged. The church figures in a particularly central way as confessional speech, a powerful normative religious discourse, is used to challenge the church's authority.

Chapter 9, the final chapter, revisits the theoretical discussions first announced in the initial chapters and developed ethnographically throughout the book. As befits a first person virtue ethics, I return to the families who have been my primary protagonists as I offer a series of epilogues or "end notes." I conclude by recounting one last funeral to ask how tragedy, critique, and moral possibility can be so intimately linked and why this ethically matters.

First Person Virtue Ethics and the Anthropology of Morality

Broadly speaking, two philosophical traditions of ethics inform current conversations about morality in anthropology. The most prominent and well known takes as its point of departure Foucault's conception of subjectivation and "care of the self." Another draws upon the Anglo-American philosophical revival of neo-Aristotelian ethics (or "virtue ethics") within ordinary language philosophy with its challenges of culture-independent moral frameworks (primarily Kantian and utilitarian ones). Sometimes these two traditions are brought together in anthropological accounts and are seen as complementary. I take a more contrarian position (for reasons I elaborate subsequently). Admittedly, there is a good deal of overlap in the two traditions. Both contest Western modernity's project to replace traditional authority with reason and to develop a procedural approach for the moral justification of a course of action. Modernity's schemes argue for principles that could be ratified by "any rational person" and thus be "independent of all those social and cultural particularities which the Enlightenment thinkers took to be the mere accidental clothing of reason in particular times and places" (MacIntyre 1988:6).

Anthropologists have long been concerned to challenge what we might think of as a (Western-inherited) ethical common sense. Modernity (meaning, roughly, the period beginning with the Enlightenment and whose ending is in controversy) has offered powerful frameworks for considering moral reasoning rooted in an understanding of rationality itself. These assumptions and frameworks continue to permeate commonsense thinking in Western societies.

For much of the discipline's life, anthropology's discussion of morality has shed a critical light upon Enlightenment universalist ideals, especially claims to objectivity, truth, and rationality. In fact, challenges to universalist constructions of rationality have arguably constituted classic anthropology's central project (Good 1994).[1]

However, the recent ethical turn in anthropology has opened up new questions about how to consider the moral. Discussions of morality continue to build upon long-standing objections to Enlightenment views but also depart from earlier positions in several crucial ways. There are substantial debates among anthropologists about these matters but there seems to be widespread agreement that at least some aspects of moral life need to be connected to freedom of moral self-making, subjectivity, and choice.[2] Laidlaw, whose 2002 essay, "For an Anthropology of Ethics and Freedom," has been an important contributor to this moral turn, argued that in order for the discipline to develop more sustained reflection on ethics anthropologists needed to find ways of "describing the possibilities of human freedom: of describing, that is, how freedom is exercised in different social contexts and cultural traditions" (311).[3]

But even when introducing something like "freedom" into the disciplinary vocabulary, anthropologists have been at pains to distance themselves from any notion of the autonomous individual who can choose her own moral destiny. This raises a key dilemma. If one wants to reject, or at least problematize, modernity's primary moral stances and its universalisms *and* continue to attend to local moralities but complicate an "unfreedom" position, where might one turn, theoretically? Is there a conceptual direction that provides a starting point for attending to moralities as contextualized, local, and traditional practices but also recognizes possibilities for moral scrutiny, reflection, and choice in cultivation of a moral self? Even, perhaps, for critique of the morally normative?

One conceptual direction is backward.

As we have seen from the previous chapter, from Western antiquity we get a very different portrait of moral practice than modernity provides. The ancients offered a picture of morality closely bound up with everyday practices of self-cultivation, the elaboration of specific technologies of moral development and—most important—an insistence on the necessity of developing a virtuous character as the basis for moral action in everyday political and social life. Aristotlean ethics, in particular, has had a long claim on moral thought. It served as a dominant moral tradition not only in premodern Europe but elsewhere, influencing Christian, Judaic, and Islamic scholars for hundreds of years.[4] Both Foucault's account of subjectivation and Anglo-American virtue ethics are deeply indebted to this ancient ethics.

It is not surprising that revisiting premodern virtue ethics of Greek and Roman antiquity has gained popularity in anthropology's contemporary ethical turn as a viable inspiration for rethinking the moral. What is *more* surprising is that one of the most central voices has been Foucault. Indeed, while anthropologists have often been leery of moral philosophy, finding philosophers largely unhelpful because they neglect to situate moral subjects in social and cultural worlds (Howell 1997), Foucault's studies are a notable exception. If Durkheim once reigned supreme in shaping anthropology's understanding of the moral, it might be argued that Foucault has now dethroned him. His work has helped to inspire an outpouring of recent anthropological studies of moral subjectivity across a broad range of social settings and practices.[5] As Faubion, an influential scholar in the new ethical turn, remarks, "Unsurprisingly, the best recent contributions to an anthropology of ethics tend to acknowledge Michel Foucault as at least one near forerunner" (2010:84). Foucault's influence bears special mention not only because he is such a central figure but also because he has inspired versions of virtue ethics that differ sharply in some grounding assumptions from a first person position.[6]

In highlighting Foucault as my key spokesperson for this contrast position and linking him so closely to a diverse constructivist tradition, I am purposely sidestepping a central feature of the Foucault legacy, namely the deeply conflicting ways that his late work is being read. Some of the most compelling recent interpretations of Foucault contend that he needs to be understood in a discontinuous way. They distance his late works on ethics from his earlier work that emphasized power and governmentality and sometimes unite him with philosophers of the "first person" sort.[7] My purpose is not to debate how Foucault's ethics should most accurately be considered. Rather, I am concerned with a *Foucauldian tradition* that interprets his late work in light of his earlier works, a tradition that continues to dominate contemporary considerations of ethics in both anthropology and cultural studies. This includes scholars who distance themselves from Foucault's earlier power/knowledge positions but continue to reject or remain wary of introducing strong notions of individual subjectivity, or a phenomenological focus on experience into their accounts.

It is this "discursive Foucault" who provides a contrast perspective from the first person framework I develop here. Throughout the book, I address lines of demarcation drawn around three key points: (1) the place of power, and critique more generally, in an account of the ethical; (2) what constitutes an appropriate conception of a moral self; and (3) the "So what?" challenge. Or, in other words, "Why does this argument matter?"

In what follows, to help clarify where a first person virtue ethics parts company with the Foucauldian discursive tradition, I take two steps. First, I further situate my framework within both phenomenology and neo-Aristotelian virtue ethics, focusing upon what has been at stake in the insistence on a first person approach to moral becoming. I do not attempt a comprehensive overview of the philosophical literature (a task well outside the purview of this book) but rather highlight those arguments most pertinent for my case. Second, I put the two positions in debate, looking with particular care at the challenges a first person ethics faces from the discursive camp.

WHAT IS FIRST PERSON VIRTUE ETHICS? A VERY SHORT PHILOSOPHY STORY

In the tradition of continental philosophy, scholars within phenomenology, hermeneutics, and existentialism were instrumental in fostering a neo-Aristotelian revival that philosophers continue to develop in various ways. Heidegger offered his contemporaries and students a new reading of Aristotle in the second and third decades of the twentieth century.[8] Heidegger came to recognize that Aristotle was not simply the "classifier" that he had been seen as but offered an avenue for grounding a practical ontology that wed hermeneutics and phenomenology to everyday practice and to a temporality of human becoming.

Historically within philosophy, a phenomenological focus on a first person perspective was not concerned with ethics as much as with contesting dominant conceptions of knowledge and ontology. Emphasizing a first person point of view challenged a portrait of knowledge that accompanied the rising authority of science in the seventeenth and eighteenth centuries. Knowledge became associated with method and privileged a certain kind of theoretical attitude: detached from everyday concerns, cool, impartial. This theoretical attitude continues to be idealized in popular belief and associated with the practice of science. What phenomenologists have argued is that this attitude also gives us a relationship to the world that presents the world to us in a particular, highly problematic kind of way. Meanings and values are abstracted from the things we study, which are then presented to us as "brute objects." As Guignon puts it, "Phenomenologists suggest that when things are seen in terms of such an objectifying point of view, the world seems to 'go dead' for us: the thick texture of meaning and values that presents itself in our everyday lives is bleached out, covered over, with the consequence that the bases of our ordinary motivation are concealed" (2009:169).

The moral implications of these insights were not always evident or of interest in the phenomenological tradition. Rather, it was the revival of Aristotle in Anglo-American moral philosophy that foregrounded the ethical. This came about several decades after Heidegger's reintroduction of Aristotle to continental philosophy—in about the middle of the twentieth century. There are many reasons for this "discovery" of Aristotle in ordinary language philosophy and philosophy of action. One is rooted in a commitment that was also part of the phenomenological project (as discussed in the previous chapter) to put forward a picture of action that could counter mechanistic or third person explanations of human action then dominant within the social and historical sciences. The basic argument was that rather than subsuming actions under general laws, one could consider them in terms of intentions and consequences—and this presumed first person agents who had reasons, desires, and some ends toward which they were fashioning their purposes.[9]

But it is in the work of such moral and political philosophers as Anscombe, Foot, MacIntyre, Taylor, Wiggins, Williams, Nussbaum, Arendt, Murdoch, and Cavell that we find a strongly marked *first person* tradition of *virtue ethics*. Beginning in the 1950s and 1960s, philosophers began to mount their own critiques of Enlightenment moral schemes, returning to Aristotelian virtue ethics for inspiration.[10] Among Anglo-American moral philosophers, virtue ethics was "initially introduced to distinguish an approach in normative ethics which emphasizes the virtues, or moral character, in contrast to an approach which emphasizes duties or rules (deontology) or one which emphasizes the consequences of action (utilitarianism)" (Hursthouse 1999:1). It is both old (because inspired by premodern moral theory) and new in the sense of emerging as one of the most recent additions to contemporary Western moral theory.

Although philosophers have often called upon it to contest crucial tenets of modernity's moral claims, virtue ethics philosophers do not speak with a unified voice. The differences among them are sufficiently marked that one notable contributor—Martha Nussbaum—once irascibly called for the term to be given up entirely to avoid confusion (Nussbaum 1999). Lines have also become blurred. Virtue ethics has become less fractiously situated vis-à-vis alternative moral theories as it has gained status in mainstream moral philosophy. Once taken seriously, it has generated new interest in the virtues among Kantians and utilitarians who are working to consider virtues in terms of their own theories. It has triggered exploration of how (previously neglected) accounts of the virtues were articulated by Enlightenment's primary moral philosophers (Nussbaum 1999). These complications notwithstanding, it is fair to say that the contemporary and predominantly Anglo-American virtue ethics tradition emphasizes distinct features of moral life disregarded or less obviously developed in the alternative moral traditions.

Most central is the importance placed on a culturally elaborated (or at least recognized) conception of the self, as mentioned in the first chapter. It is in the name of such a self that virtue ethicists have mounted a commonly shared critique of modernity's primary alternatives, arguing that these traditions tend to leave out or flatten consideration of motives and moral character as well as a host of other important considerations that recognize the concrete situatedness of moral action and the intimate social relatedness of our moral concerns. This content filled and psychologically complex moral agent is firmly located in particular cultural and historical settings, a picture that contrasts sharply with the detached or universalized moral agent associated with modernity's moral schemes (Lear 2006). In the first chapter, I emphasized the importance of narrative to this revival of virtue ethics; a narrative conception of the self has seemed to many philosophers a requirement of any such thick depiction.

In its revival, contemporary theorists have discarded many of the parochial assumptions characterizing that Athenian-inspired worldview, particularly its notorious views on women and slavery. Also, some of the virtues held in most esteem by the Athenians (like courage) or neglected (like benevolence) have routinely been revised by contemporary moral theorists. Its attraction, generally, has been its ability to address qualities of moral life disregarded by the two primary alternatives, not only "motives and moral character" but also "moral education, moral wisdom or discernment, friendship and family relationships, a deep concept of happiness, the role of the emotions in our moral life, and the questions of what sort of person I should be and of how we should live" (Hursthouse 1999:3).

Intriguingly, while male philosophers have been significant contributors, a number of influential female philosophers were crucial voices from the start; an essay by Oxford philosopher Anscombe (1958) is generally credited with the reintroduction of this tradition into philosophical thought. It is no great wonder that in the revival of virtue ethics, which owes much to female and feminist-friendly philosophers, *care of others* and the domestic sphere of intimate familial relationships often serve as exemplars for considering the complexities and challenges of moral life.[11] (This, it goes without saying, was not the sphere that Aristotle had in mind, with his emphasis on the public space of the "polis.") Feminist literature has sometimes drawn upon this work to promote a care ethics that privileges a "connected self" rather than an autonomous one and stresses responsibilities, relationships, intersubjectivity, the circumstantiality of ethics and activity rather than rules and abstract reasoning (Tronto 1993).

Philosophy's virtue ethics provides conceptual support for a historically and culturally shaped understanding of ethics grounded in social practice. Although virtue ethics philosophers have often been concerned to avoid moral relativism (e.g., Nussbaum 1999), the insistence on socially situated moral agents bears a fortuitous kinship with anthropology's longstanding mission to repudiate modernity's aspiration to get beyond the "accidental trappings" of morality. A virtue ethics portrait of the moral as related to practices of cultivating virtue also resonates with anthropological studies of how the moral is *learned* and negotiated in important domains such as the family.[12] As Laidlaw points out, there is a natural affinity between the anthropological value of creating what Geertz has called "thick description" and the virtue ethicists' recognition that an adequate moral psychology demands a cultural approach, even an "ethnographic stance" (Williams 1986:203–4, cited in Laidlaw 2013:47). This is not an accidental affinity. Geertz creatively drew upon philosophy in his own interpretive theory, including the Oxford philosophers who were so instrumental in articulating their own versions of morally "thick descriptions" of character and agency (Mattingly and Jensen, in press).

Despite differences in vocabulary and perspective, both the continental and Anglo-American first person traditions share a commitment to articulate a practice-based ethics that bears an allegiance to a certain form of humanism or is, at least, anti-anti-humanist. But to say that they are humanist requires further clarification, because the term *humanism* can stand for many things. I emphasize particularly their resonance with a premodern sensibility (especially as expressed by the Greek dramatists) in which persons are not considered autonomous individuals but vulnerable social creatures, dependent upon circumstances often out of human control and certainly out of control of the singular moral agent.

From the Enlightenment on, humanism—reflections on what it is to be human—comes to mean something very different. It becomes associated with secularism and moral autonomy. It offers what Charles Taylor has called a "self sufficing humanism" that rejects any spiritual or cosmological vision of reality and foregrounds the free and singular moral agent. In the moral frameworks that belong to modernity, in other words, humans are the apex of any hierarchy of being. The humanism of the ancients differs radically in this respect. There was always some sense of a higher order, one that was beyond or above human life. In this sense, as Taylor argues, Aristotle shared more of a worldview with contemporary religious communities than with modernity or any postmodernisms:

> The general understanding of the human predicament before modernity placed us in an order where we were not at the top. Higher beings, like Gods or spirits, or a higher kind of being, like the Ideas or the cosmopolis of Gods and humans, demanded and deserved our worship, reference, devotion or love. In some cases, this reverence or devotion was itself seen as integral to human flourishing; it was a proper part of the human good. . . . [Thus] we might speak of a humanism, but not of a self-sufficing or exclusive humanism. (Taylor 2007:18–19)

The "exclusive humanism" of modernity, Taylor asserts, is not only to be contrasted with premodern philosophies or religions but also with what he labels "non-religious anti-humanisms, which fly under various names today, like 'deconstruction' and 'post-structuralism'" (2007:19).

Taylor is positing that humans are necessarily relational and relationships can, of course, include nonhuman beings like gods or spirits. However, this relational primacy does not negate the idea of an individual's historical particularity as shaped by the singularities of circumstances and commitments. In fact, it is just this particularity that many virtue ethicists have sought to emphasize. Bernard Williams, for example, asserts that it is precisely because our relationships with others are so important to us that some concept of moral individuality is required. For Williams, cultivating moral character is intertwined with a person's commitments to particular ground projects and these include his relations with specific other individuals. The whole notion of character gives "substance to the idea that individuals are not inter-substitutable" (1981:15). Friendship provides a telling illustration. "To the thought that his friend cannot just be equivalently replaced by another friend, is added both the thought that he cannot just be replaced himself, and also the thought that he and his friend are different from each other" (1981:15). Although Williams offers a more secular argument than Taylor's, both insist that ethics requires individual (but not autonomous) selves for any adequate moral account.

VIRTUE ETHICS IN DEBATE

I have organized the remainder of this chapter as a kind of quarrel. My dialogical strategy is to consider some important critiques that confront a first person framework, offering brief rebuttals to these objections. I also tackle a different kind of challenge, one that questions this whole debating enterprise. This might be called the "So what?" complaint. One could reasonably contend that scholarly positions and voices need not be wholly consistent to be usable in ethnography because we anthropologists develop theory in another way. (Leave that to the philosophers!) One could also note the many convergences among these two ethics traditions and decide that it makes more sense to pay attention to what they share than how they diverge. Furthermore, one might point out, there are numerous ways a first person position is already entailed in ethnographic description; therefore it needs no theoretical defense or elaboration. My general response here is that the schisms in the current conversation deserve to be named and explored, as indeed, a number of anthropologists have been doing along various lines (e.g., Fassin 2008; Faubion 2011; Laidlaw 2013; Mattingly 2012; Robbins 2007, 2009; Stoczkowski 2008; Yan 2011; Zigon 2008, 2009). My refutations are schematic in this chapter; the strength of my position ultimately depends upon the chapters that follow in which abstract arguments are elaborated in ethnographic context using detailed examples.

First Challenge: The Power/Critical Theory Objection

One of the great attractions of Foucault is that his work has made it possible to connect moral subjectivity to power in illuminating ways that other philosophical moral frameworks—and certainly neo-Aristotelian virtue ethics—do not seem to provide. It is well known that

Foucault was long interested in the moral, and especially the pernicious ways moral claims were made (against the mad, the criminal, and other deviants) as part of "rehabilitative" practices that constructed those very categories and created new forms of knowledge that defined them. Foucault has had enormous influence on anthropological theorizing about modern modes of governmentality and the insidious work of bureaucratic power in shaping docile bodies.

But it is Foucault's late work (primarily the final two books in the *History of Sexuality* series but also his final interviews and lectures) that has currently commanded widespread attention, allowing a wide range of readings about self-cultivation as a moral project. His investigation of ancient Greek and Roman ethical thought was key to the development of his ethics of self-care. Foucault's work has helped introduce virtue ethics to a broad audience outside philosophy. As he pointed out, from the perspective of antiquity, moral action could not be disassociated from a whole mode of being, a mode of life and a relationship to the self. It was not reducible to conforming to a rule or a law but flows from an entire process of self-formation as an "ethical subject." In one of his most often-cited quotes he defined the moral domain in the following way. It designated

> *a process in which the individual delimits that part of himself that will form the object of his moral practice, defines his position relative to the precept he will follow, and decides on a certain mode of being that will serve as his moral goal. And this requires him to act upon himself, to monitor, test, improve and transform himself. There is no specific moral action that does not refer to a unified moral conduct; no moral conduct that does not call for the forming of oneself as an ethical subject; and no forming of the ethical subject without "modes of subjectivation" and an "ascetics" or "practices of the self" that support them. Moral action is indissociable from these forms of self-activity.* (1990b)

Foucault introduced an avenue for considering ethics that seemed to offer a way out of a conceptual impasse, making it possible to steer clear of modernity's Archimedean portrayals of moral choice (the view from nowhere) while avoiding cultural historical determinisms. It suggested that the ethical could be understood as the freedom to choose *which* kind of ethical regime (among the available varieties) one could subject oneself to, a freedom that was formed within and shaped by the cultural communities one inhabited.[13]

For many scholars, this formulation is particularly useful precisely because it offers new ways to link ethical self-formation to power. While

Foucault's discussion of self-care as self-reliance in his later works may seem at odds with his earlier work on the disciplining of bodies and the role of expertise in disciplinary power (and may be treated as such by contemporary scholars), it is also plausible to read his late work as still calling upon the insights and framework that informed his earlier thinking. The requirement to care for oneself also entails putting oneself in the care of experts who will guide that care. Self-care and this expert care go hand in hand. In fact, the strong cultural belief that "care of the self" is a moral obligation can also promote an increasing exercise of expert power in just those situations in which designated populations—say the insane or the criminal—are deemed morally incapable of directing their own self-care.

Even in his late work, Foucault often contended that the kinds of power dynamics that rested upon technologies of domination could be, and generally were, intertwined with technologies of self.[14] While Foucault certainly provides a means for talking about moral practice, moral self-mastery, and the cultivation of virtues, he offers a position that readily lends itself to recognizing how easily moral practices of self-cultivation can be no more than (or less than) practices of normalization within a particular regime of truth. Foucault's considerations of the moral, particularly when wedded to his analyses of biopower and governmentality, have proved enormously fruitful. They have generated a host of anthropological studies that eschew any robust first person perspective on the grounds that this mislocates the true source of agency (which is structural) and has the unfortunate consequence of "blaming the victim" by ascribing freedoms to individual actors that are a mere mirage. This is a serious and important objection, especially for a virtue ethics that has such close ties to Aristotle. After all, from our contemporary vantage point, Aristotle must be considered not only parochial but elitist.

In short, here is the challenge as I see it: How can we make a case for taking seriously just those claims to first person moral experience and projects of moral becoming that those we study take seriously but also preserve the important insights of discursive critical theories, especially concerning the (often insidious and masked) role of social structures in forming selves?

Second Challenge: The "Death of the Self" Objection

Put most bluntly, the objection goes something like this: The whole notion of the "individual" or the "experiencing self" is an erroneous humanist construction that should be abandoned except when treated merely as an "effect" of discursive traditions and structural forces. Much more is at play here than the familiar agency/structure debate. This challenge is so consequential that I spend considerable time outlining it. There is a significant history that explains why the rejection of a first person self is so compelling and why first person accounts are so difficult to reconcile with alternative poststructural approaches. The poststructuralist enterprise has been concerned to expose and dismantle some of the key concepts associated with humanism, especially the notion of an "I" and a "we" who are a locus of agency, experience, the unity of a life—precisely the heart of first person perspectives. In *The Postmodern Condition* (1979), Lyotard offered his famously influential "death of the subject" proclamations. He wrote dismissively of modernity's misguided belief in experience that presupposed "the instance of an 'I' who speaks in the first person" and "temporal arrangements" of past, present, and future—a kind of narrative coherence of the self, in other words. The interrelated terms—*experience, the first person perspective,* and a *temporal self*—were seen as an unfortunate product of Christianity and its model of salvation.[15] The problematizing of "experience" has been crucial not only among those who are concerned that it obscures the focus on the discursive, economic, and political, but even among anthropology's phenomenologists. Desjarlais, for example, has suggested that "experience" as commonly associated with a self who coheres over time is not an "existential given" but one human possibility among others (2010:161), and he situates the emergence of this enduring, experiencing self within a very specific European history (see also Desjarlais 1996, 1997).

Such radical doubts pose a problem not only for a first person virtue ethics but, more broadly, for anthropologists who want to speak, analytically, about first person individuals. Caroline Humphrey puts it this way: "Certain kinds of anthropological experience seem to require the conceptualization of singular analytical subjects: individual actors who are constituted as subjects in particular circumstances" (2008:357). But it has become quite difficult these days to offer such subjects. The difficulty, Humphrey points out, "lies in the fact that 'the death of the subject' has been convincingly argued for in so many disciplines in the humanities and social sciences ... [that] it is no longer possible to assume the simple presence of 'the individual subject,' as if that idea had not already been radically undermined by generations of philosophers and anthropologists of the 20th century."

In trying to understand what it means to have a self, Foucauldian discursive accounts direct us to ask, What kind of an "I" is created in particular historical and cultural conditions? That is, what kinds of subjects are produced? What are the normative technologies at work in shaping subjectivities? (e.g., Butler 2005) Poststructuralists tend to characterize as naïve or essentialist any conceptual versions of an "I" that do *not* presuppose this primary interrogation. Initially this was the charge made by Foucault and other young poststructuralists to the Sartrean existentialism that dominated the philosophical milieu of postwar France (Flynn 1997), but their critique was intended to encompass the broader array of phenomenological and hermeneutic traditions, as well as the moral schemes of Enlightenment. Here, the whole family of humanist first person terms (e.g., self, agency, experience, motive, self-interpretation) are carefully excised, or rather, more precisely, redefined as the *effects* of collective practices. Notably, this expunging often involves an identification of humanism solely with the Enlightenment moral project, as when Mahmood identifies "the legacy of humanist ethics" primarily with "its Kantian formulation" (2005:119).

Nikolas Rose (1998) offers an especially decisive condemnation of just those constructs that first person humanist ethics requires. Rose points to poststructuralist writing that has finally exposed the "death of the self." He notes with approval the many theorists who have offered us "countless obituaries of the image of the human being that animated our philosophies and our ethics for so long, a subject that is stable, unified, totalized, individualized, interiorized" (1998:169). From Rose's point of view, this portrait has been so thoroughly demolished that it is simply untenable to hold onto it any longer. But he notices, in everyday life, that this portrait flourishes more than ever as "regulatory practice seeks to govern individuals in a way more tied to their 'selfhood' than ever before" (1998:169). In a whole range of practices, including medicine and health, he notes, "human beings are addressed, represented, and acted upon *as if they were selves* of a particular type: suffused with an individual subjectivity, motivated by anxieties and aspirations concerning their self-fulfillment, committed to finding their true identities and maximizing their authentic expressions in their lifestyles" (1998:169–70). Equally in our political thinking, we "operate in terms of an image of each human being as the unified psychological focus of his or her biography" (1998:170). Rose suggests that ordinary practices continue to be based upon these erroneous presumptions of an interior, coherent, agentive self, revealing how everyday persons are not only in the grip of this cultural mystification, but that such common sense ideas about free-dom and selfhood make a troublesome neoliberal government possible.

At a theoretical level, differences between a Foucauldian discursive and a neo-Aristotelian first person positions may seem immense. But from an anthropological and more practical fieldwork level in which we ask such questions as "What does a conceptual framework allow us to see and what does it hide?," the differences between these positions are more subtle. Conceptually, too, in terms of clearly articulated positions, things are often blurrier. A fundamental or un-worked-out set of controversies seems to plague the anthropology of morality concerning the status of the self. What exactly is meant by a "self" here? Is this the "self" consistent with the one presumed by most first person ethics philosophers? One who has some agentive powers, is capable of self-reflection, interpretation, and critique of moral norms? Or is this self best understood as a product of a particular cultural, historical milieu—a self-identified by its subject position? In other words, is this moral self best thought of as an *effect* of the moral practices, traditions, and technologies in which it has been enculturated?

The latter view is especially congruent with prevailing anthropological thought that has always been wary of too much individualism, emphasizing the cultural and structural production of selves. Current Foucauldian-inspired inquiries into biosociality, biopower, and govern-mentality continue to accentuate this perspective. However, because anthropologists have also tried to make some room for moral freedom and moral deliberation and have turned to Foucault as a support for this, it is not always clear whether or not they are also adopting some version of a first person self more congruent with neo-Aristotelian virtue ethics.

Given that Foucault has been such an important contributor to recent discussions, it is plausible to suppose that this anthropological muddi-ness reflects an inconsistency in Foucault's own evolving (or discontinu-ous?) thinking. In Foucault's late work, when he offers a virtue ethics based upon Hellenistic and Roman developments of Platonic and Aris-totelian thought, he sometimes seems to be embracing some form of an agentive first person self. However, many scholars would argue that even in Foucault's "return to the Greeks" (Levy 2004:20), he continues to repudiate the more fully fleshed out and "thick" kind of first person self that most contemporary virtue ethics philosophers would insist upon. In Paras's careful account, he argues that Foucault introduces an unresolved confusion. In his most influential earlier work, especially *Discipline and Punish*, subjectivity is the product of techniques rather than, as he suggests later, a target of techniques. But these imply contradictory positions. Paras puts the dilemma as follows: "If subjectivity is the *target* of techniques rather than the *product* of techniques, then we are entitled to wonder where that subjectivity comes from in the first place. . . . When he continued to claim, and perhaps to believe, that he was describing the construction of subjects through discourse, his arguments told otherwise" (2006:123, emphasis added).

Usefully, for my heuristic purposes, some anthropologists have offered clear and subtly developed repudiations of an analytically consequential first person self, strongly distinguishing their kind of moral self from a robust first person position. I call upon two of them to help clarify differences. Divergences emerge most significantly around the question of the *locus of ethical agency*. The first person position privileges both the "we" (first person plural) and the "I" (first person singular) as primary sites of ethical practice, though always understood as existing within histories that precede any "I" or "we." Third person or discursive positions contrastively favor systems, social practices, or the technologies within particular "regimes of truth" (to borrow Foucault's language) as the primary agentive sites. Generally speaking, when anthropologists turn to Foucauldian traditions, they foreground the shared practices, technologies, and discourses that form ethical subjectivity. This focus presumes that personal ethical subjectivity can largely be explained by these powerful preexisting moral codes and practices.

Saba Mahmood's study of women's participation in Islamic religious practices provides a compelling example. She offers an expanded understanding of agency that counters a familiar feminist portrait in which agency is identified with resistance to hegemonic systems of power. By tackling the question of ethical agency, Mahmood might seem to depend upon a first person "I" in her account of moral agency. But not so. Her clear and explicit dismissal of this "I" is instructive. She, in fact, worries that although she has explicitly rejected humanism (which she characterizes as presuming a "sovereign subject") in drawing upon Foucault's work on ethical self-formation, she might mistakenly appear to have "smuggled back in a subject-centered theory of agency by locating agency within the efforts of the self" (2005:32). She addresses this potential misunderstanding by further distancing herself from any notion of the individual as agent. "The kind of agency I am exploring," she tells us, "does not belong to the women themselves, but is a product of the historically contingent discursive traditions in which they are located" (2005:32). Thus, work on the ethical self is a matter of being interpellated, being "summoned" to "recognize [oneself] in terms of the virtues and codes" of particular traditions (2005:32). It is this process that her ethnography elaborates. She articulates and develops a picture of virtue ethics that foregrounds the "specific sets of procedures, techniques, and exercises through which highly specific ethical-moral subjects come to be formed" (2005:120).

As illustrated by Mahmood's exposition, a robust first person ethical tradition is challenged by one that emphasizes the pedagogical nature of becoming a certain sort of ethical subject *when* such becoming is equated with, as Faubion puts it, "striving toward the occupancy of a 'subject position'" (2011:4). In their very different ways, both Faubion and Mahmood emphasize how deeply moral subjectivity and selfhood are structurally embedded within prearticulated conceptions of the good; the *telos* of one's ethical striving is defined in advance by the moral good that is attached to a particular subject position. To continue with Faubion's reading for a moment more: "Indefinitely many actors might strive toward the same telos; indefinitely many of them might thus end up being the same subject, if with idiosyncratic variations from one case to another" (2011:4). From this perspective, the differences that distinguish one subject from another can reasonably be described in the manner he does—as "idiosyncratic variations."

Faubion's framework is particularly illuminating because he shows us how a first person self can be dismissed even in an ethnobiographical account of moral subjectivity. He introduces his life history chapters of *An Anthropology of Ethics* with the following declaration: "To reiterate: neither methodologically nor ontologically does an anthropology of ethics have its ground in the individual. The population of its interpretive universe is instead one of subjects in or passing through positions in environments" (2011:119). Faubion's notion of the ethical subject offers a compelling contrast with a first person perspective. What is important here is not simply that Faubion is insistent upon resisting some kind of methodological or ontological individualism (as would first person virtue ethicists) but that he is prepared to include as ethical subjects entities he would also call "objects." As he goes on to say, this population called the "ethical subject" could just as well include "human collectives, or even human and non-human collectives or assemblages of one or another kind. Nothing in principle precludes the possibility of a cyborgic ethics, an ethics of quasi-objects" (2011:119).

This intellectual move makes sense if being an ethical subject means, first and foremost, inhabiting a particular social location, or more precisely, as Faubion puts it, "passing through positions in environments."

However, something like "quasi-objects" are not possible candidates for moral subjects within first person virtue ethics, in which the first person human (singular and plural) is the primary moral subject. Contemporary first person virtue ethics, in other words, though rejecting ideas of autonomous individuals or a "self-sufficing humanism" that necessarily excludes, say, gods or other spirits, does call upon a vocabulary surrounding the ethical subject that includes such features as motives, self-interpretation, reflection, embodied experience, and the like. The first person character of this version means that it does not include, as ethical subjects, something we would call "objects."

I have offered examples from some well-known scholars to make my point but, speaking more generally, we can see how a first person ethics faces the serious problem of being associated not only with a questionable Christian-based humanism but an unsophisticated descriptive phenomenology. Strategies to distance oneself from such theoretical perspectives continue to be an important concern for many anthropologists where the individual has always been "intellectually unfashionable" (Jackson 1996:23).[16] A first person self is even more unfashionable for those scholars who posit not only "discursive subjects" but also "quasi-subjects," "partible persons," or various types of agents composed of nonhuman and human parts.

Third Challenge: "So What?" Why Does This Argument Matter?

In very broad strokes, I have outlined two contrasting pictures of virtue ethics, one dependent upon a "thick" first person moral self, and one (usually grounded in poststructuralisms of various stripes) largely hostile to this idea. I have also stressed points of difference. But, one could object, why should anthropologists care? This may be another matter better left to philosophers, a scholastic squabble that can safely be ignored. Because so many anthropologists have found their way into virtue ethics primarily through Foucault rather than hermeneutic, phenomenological, or ordinary language philosophy,[17] philosophical quarrels may be unfamiliar or seem not especially relevant. Also, when we turn to search out ethnographies explicitly developing a first person tradition, things get blurrier. Certainly there are no "strictly speaking" neo-Aristotelian anthropologists, just as there are (probably) no "strictly speaking" Foucauldian (or Deleuzian or Latourian, etc.) ones.

Furthermore, as already noted, there are a number of points of overlap between a first person ethics and a poststructural one, especially when drawing upon Foucault. Both have positioned themselves critically vis-à-vis Enlightenment moral frameworks. Both are in broad sympathy with anthropological critiques of universal reason. That is, both claim that a moral decision or action cannot be determined through some universal set of rules, procedures, or reasoning processes that one derives from an Archimedean position. Rather, the moral is always historical, always shaped by social context. (Though what *context* comes to mean is very different in these two traditions.) Both contend that the moral in any society is dependent upon the cultivation of virtues that are developed in and through social practices. For both, the moral is centrally bound up with practices of self-care and self-cultivation; it is not captured by espoused beliefs but rather involves the emotions, the body, everyday activity. It is an integral and pervasive aspect of social life. Both frameworks also emphasize that the moral is a communal enterprise; there are no persons here who are independent of the practical communities that shape the technologies of virtue and the aspirations about the good life to which individuals ascribe.

Based upon these points of intersection, it is very tempting to imagine that a Foucauldian and a first person position on ethics could not only be blended but could provide a corrective to the other. Foucault gives first person Aristotelians a vehicle for paying serious attention to the discursive structures that shape how the moral is framed, thus locating the moral within the cultural and historical in a way that brings in politics and the history of discourses into the frame. First person ethics, with its focus on situated action, on practice as experienced, and on the moral deliberation of individuals acting within communities, brings agency, experience, and motive into focus, enriching our understanding of the moral dimensions of lived experience and social action.

Perhaps the most significant factor that makes it so intuitive to treat these ethical frameworks as complementary rather than competing has to do with how anthropologists do their research. Most essentially, there is the matter of the sheer thickness, the nuance, of ethnographic examples. The methods of anthropology produce slices of the world that overflow, elide, slip away from the systematic purity of theory. This penchant for messiness is no accident; in fact its production in field notes and monographs is a matter of some disciplinary pride. Part of the job of the anthropologist in the field is to undergo a form of immersion in some local reality (or realities), compelling her to rethink, modify, or even discard the theoretical frameworks she has learned. This is not because theory is without merit. It is simply because theory, being general, cannot be expected to capture the subtlety of the particular events that the fieldworker is documenting. In an effort to do justice to this kind of phenomenal complexity, the anthropologist may draw upon a variety of theorists, but the field itself—the people, the events, the experiences that the anthropologist has—all this messy "reality" (for want of a better term)—is *expected to talk back*. It is expected to resist, to surprise, to call for new questions, to undo assumptions. This is the hope and the challenge of the anthropological method.

Furthermore, no matter what their theoretical predilections, most anthropologists continue to do ethnography of a recognizable participant observation sort. That is, they engage in a kind of research practice that involves them in "experience-near" encounters with particular people they come to know over time. In general, they continue to investigate how people living within given social communities produce, traverse, and make sense of those worlds. They continue, in other words, to try to access indigenous first person perspective(s) on life as lived by particular people. As a result, even when they adopt third person social theories as primary explanatory frameworks, this does not obviate the very first person approach that ethnographic research continues to call for.

One consequence of the culture critique leveled in the 1980s is that anthropologists, wary of making problematic claims about homogeneous, timeless cultural wholes, have increasingly foregrounded the particularity of individuals living under historically specific social conditions. Life histories are a common tool for examining how some social world is inhabited and (to speak in familiar poststructural terms) its varieties of subject positions embodied and performed. Anthropology's first person style of study makes it not only possible but perhaps inevitable that the *descriptive passages* of ethnographies concerned with moral life—what we might think of as ethnography's empirical (but not empiricist) heart—will represent the moral, at least in part, in first person terms. Additionally, anthropologists bring their own first person perspectives to their research encounters and the presence of the anthropologist continues to be marked in contemporary ethnographies. The influence of the reflexive turn within the discipline that began in the 1970s and 1980s can still be felt; texts often include brief autobiographical forays. The need for such reflexivity has been recently voiced around worries that an anthropology of morality might become synonymous with self-righteous moralizing (Stoczkowski 2008; Zigon 2007, 2008). Fassin argues that the only protection from such moralism (especially when studying oppressed peoples) is for the anthropologist to consider his "own moral prejudices . . . as objects of his scientific investigation as well as those of his 'others'"(2008: 337).

If we anthropologists engage first person perspectives on the moral in all these ways, why can't we use our theoretical efforts to embed the individual particularities and idiosyncracies of our informants (and ourselves) within large-scale discursive frameworks? Why isn't it sufficient to use life narratives as vantage points for representing how selves are interpellated and subject positions performed, thus giving our work greater theoretical muscle and reach? Why, in other words, haven't anthropologists managed to solve a problem that philosophers continue to wrestle with precisely through this kind of division of intellectual labor?

To make matters more confusing, anthropologists concerned to further a critique of dominant structures of power may at times develop decidedly Foucauldian approaches to governmentality while at other times articulate positions much more compatible with first person virtue ethics or simply interweave the two. For example, anthropologists drawing upon phenomenology and other theories of subjectivity have not only investigated how lived experience is shaped by a variety of particular social, cultural, and political forces, foregrounding its social, historical, and intersubjective nature, but also added a critical and historical dimension that owes a large debt to Foucault. This has entailed efforts to simultaneously trace the "genealogy" of what it means to be a subject—especially a "modern subject"—in a more third person historical manner and attend to the particular experiences of individuals (e.g., Biehl, Good, and Kleinman 2007). These efforts reflect anthropology's long-standing concern not to reduce experience or subjectivity to an individualist psychology and to search for ways to theorize agency that do not leave structural and cultural conditions behind (Luhrmann 2006; Ortner 2005; Zigon 2011). In this vein, many phenomenological approaches in anthropology now offer variations of what Desjarlais (1996, 1997) has called "critical phenomenology."[18]

In light of all this, my attempt to distinguish two versions of virtue ethics might seem so much scholastic nonsense, just the sort of stuffy in-fighting and crankiness one can expect from the Academy.

Rebuttals

These are three substantial challenges that are not readily dismissed. How might they be addressed? The initial challenge (What about power and governmentality?) is a concern shared by many neo-Aristotelians, especially those focused on social justice. I often call upon their reworkings in the chapters that follow. As a number of them have pointed out, the importance even in ancient Athens of being able to critique the commonsense wisdom of the day was essential to the philosophical mission and embedded in civil society. The notion of "truth telling" that Foucault takes up in his final works is inspired by this ancient tradition of critique.

But it is not enough to notice that there were traditions of critiques in other, earlier times. What is added by investigating social critique in ethnographic context by drawing upon a first person framework, as I propose to do? My response is to consider critique as a first person enterprise. I consider how people strive for a good life, are plagued by moral tragedy and cultivate their own local, indigenous hermeneutics of suspicion as well as hope. All of this draws upon cultural resources. Sometimes it is expressed as an overt kind of political resistance to normative structures. But it *also* arises because of singular experiences and moral challenges people face, ones that impel them to critically evaluate and try to transcend their current situations in creative ways that are not best understood in political terms. Creative efforts at transformation encompass such a wide range of social and personal projects.

I ask, What are the resources for indigenous cultural critiques? When and under what circumstances are these called upon? How does a small experiment entail an act of social criticism? In asking such questions, it quickly becomes clear that a critically informed first person ethics (such as I try to develop here) is by no means a straightforward adoption of any conceptual approach. Instead, I follow a path typical of anthropology where one does not simply "apply" theory to one's ethnographic material but rather puts it in dialogue with that material and the social communities in which one has been immersed. Indeed, as I try to show throughout, my fieldwork among African American families and their ways of understanding their moral situations and predicaments necessitates amending and elaborating the philosophical arguments I draw upon. In the ethnographic chapters to follow, I work to articulate an ethics that incorporates some of the strengths we find in discursive style critical approaches without adopting an a priori rejection of the first person experiencing self.

The second objection, concerning the status of the experiencing self, is even more troublesome. Any first person ethics is faced with this history of skeptical repudiations of something like a "humanist individual" as well as by the new quasi-object candidates for moral subjects. If we add this to the complaints of Foucauldian governmentality theorists, the challenge could be stated as follows: Can we reassemble the self and give some room for the singularity of events and experiences while also honoring some of the insights of critical theory, including critical theory that has also radically problematized notions of self, experience, and the like?

In philosophy, this has often provoked strong debate. There has characteristically been a deep conceptual antagonism between genealogical camps and first person virtue ethics. Despite sharing many common critiques of Enlightenment moral traditions, "the different grounds from which they make that diagnosis involve each in a rejection of the other," MacIntyre argues (1990:204). One can see this in the following exchange between Charles Taylor and a Foucauldian philosopher that took place in the mid-1980s when Foucault's work on the ethics of self-care was garnering major attention. Taylor was asked to defend why he could still work on theories of moral agency and the self after Foucault. His challenger put it this way: "Foucault's theory of power and subjectification is part of his assault on those teleological philosophies that continue to find disguised expression in the modern age. The theory of the essentially embodied subject, for instance, is a theory of self-realization that treats the self as if it were designed to fulfill its potentiality through perfecting its subjectivity" (Connolly 1985:371).

Charles Taylor responded by noting that while he very much agreed with Foucault in rejecting Enlightenment ideals of universal subjects and corresponding notions of truth, he wondered why this entailed abandoning the work of developing a "hermeneutic understanding of truth as self interpretations" (1985: 385). He asked, Why does this unmasking genealogical effort somehow foreclose our continued thinking through what it meant to be a moral agent? In fact, it is just here that the real debate ought to start, he argued. As he pointed out, his own philosophical project, which has depended upon a notion of a first person moral agent, did not seem "to be in worse shape than its obvious rivals, certainly not [worse] than the Nietzchean notion of truth as imposition" (1985:385). What was needed instead, Taylor announced, was continued discussion between these rival positions and their presumptions about the self, looking at the costs of each. That is, what was to be gained or lost by holding one position rather than the other?

Although there may be no satisfying way to persuade those who are a priori committed to rejecting a first person self, it is useful—as Taylor does with his opponent—to point out the costs of this intellectual move. This is a question we might ask in light of our own ethnographic projects and concerns. Caroline Humphrey offers a penetrating consideration. She points out that the disbursement of the individual self into discursive fields, dividuals, or actor-networks presents us with a real problem. Having theoretically dispensed with the individual subject, what do we do about the fact that "as anthropologists . . . we need to be able to give an account of 'what happened', one that does not dissolve into a processual-relational haze, nor resort to explaining only the underlying conditions in which such a happening might occur (as if it could *not* have been otherwise)" (2008:358; my emphasis added). She adds a further difficulty. This concerns our own faithfulness to the people we study, for, as she points out, speaking of the Mongolian people she writes about, "they do speak constantly of singular subjects and their deeds. They talk of the consequences of someone's, a named person's, actions" (2008:358).

Humphrey's complaints might seem to be resolvable within a discursive scheme. Simply recognize that these Mongolians turn out to "speak of singular subjects and their deeds" and that this reflects one discursive possibility in the ethnographic record, among others. But this solution carries a significant cost: a systematic *undertheorizing* of first person moral perspectives within anthropology, especially as they illuminate the complexities of moral judgment and action in everyday life. This is not only important for theoretical clarity but also because it is very easy for a first person ethics to become swallowed up into its poststructuralist counterparts, thereby losing some of the most crucial insights that it has to offer. The strength of first person virtue ethics is that it attends not only to the practices of moral apprenticeship and pedagogy but also to the problem of action itself, to the *doing* of ordinary life. It directs us to what Lambek (2010b) calls "ordinary ethics,"[19] where the moral involves the exercise of practical judgment about the "best good" within the particularities of circumstances.[20] Everyday life emerges as a site of "moral striving" (Das 2010).

To investigate these aspects of moral action and experience, discursive accounts are problematic, at least as a starting point. A more useful conceptual platform must be more inclusive. It must not only foreground inherited moral traditions and already articulated practices of subjectivation. It must be equally attentive to processes of ethical judgment grounded in singular events and the formation of selves who have some agentive resilience. This means revising some very basic a priori assumptions that have been part of the discursive project and its historic rejection not only of Enlightenment moral schemes but also of first person traditions that have been central to the contemporary neo-Aristotelian revival.

I have taken an entire chapter to argue this basic point because first person ethics is far less well articulated in social theory than its discursive alternatives are. Phenomenological anthropology, an obvious starting place, is helpful but only takes us so far. Anthropologists within this tradition have insisted that one must try to assess what it means experientially to inhabit a particular lifeworld. For many, a phenomenological position assumes that we take people's own commitments and understandings of their situations into consideration in a primary way.[21] Phenomenological anthropologists have also put forward various critiques of third person explanatory schemes that downplay or exclude first person ones, making the case for the "experience near,"[22] for the moral as an experience,[23] for "radical empiricism,"[24] and, of course, "embodiment."[25] These approaches presume a strongly marked first person perspective that supports part of my proposal.[26]

However, many phenomenological anthropologists would balk at a central claim I have advanced, the analytic necessity of positing the individual as one crucial "site" of experience. It is perfectly possible to consider experience from a phenomenological first person perspective without attending to the particularity of these first persons in any analytic detail—and indeed, this may often be preferred. Douglas Hollan points this out in a remarkably clarifying discussion with anthropological phenomenology.[27] Hollan notes that although this work has been enormously useful in theorizing a variety of lifeworlds and how they are intersubjectively lived, it has been less successful in capturing how particular individuals become attuned to these lifeworlds, or how they inhabit and shape them in their own biographically particular ways. Hollan states:

> Ironically ... what seems to be missing from some of this phenomenologically inspired work is how given individuals become dynamically 'coupled with' or 'attuned to' their 'immediate' environments—that is, how they become marked by a particular set of historically specific interactions with others, and in turn, how historically specific individuals come to mark and infuse, in particular ways, the lives of others. (2012:42)

As a remedy for this neglect, Hollan builds upon anthropology's person-centered tradition, advocating an approach that draws from contemporary psychoanalysis. I am alternatively suggesting that the moral frameworks developed within first person virtue ethics offer a rich vocabulary for considering humans as "self-interpreting" moral beings whose perceptions, interpretations, and actions help shape moral subjectivities in the singular as well as the collective. Mine is not only a call to attend to the biographical specificities of given individuals (though it is that) but also an argument that we need further tools to conceptually strengthen our ways to consider moral subjectivity and its formation.

My rebuttal to the third (So what?) objection could be summed up by this call and this argument. The persuasiveness of my response will need to be assessed in light of the ethnographic chapters that follow. In these chapters, beginning with the following one, I will also respond to an additional issue and line of demarcation, the status of the moral ordinary.

PART TWO

Moral Becoming and the Everyday

CHAPTER 3

Home Experiments

Scenes from the Moral Ordinary

"Straggle" had an invented meaning—not just to stray, as the dictionary would have it, but to struggle, strive, and drag all at once. This, in my translation, meant the constant work of valuing oneself and others, of persevering against the odds, of imagining a better future and making your way, steadily, toward it.

—(Referring to a word traditionally used among African American slave women) (Miles 2008:101–2)

The fact that man is capable of action means that the unexpected can be expected from him, that he is able to perform what is infinitely improbable.

—(Arendt 1958:178)

ORDINARY LIFE AND THE ETHICAL SELF

What is this thing called "the ordinary" or "everyday life"? How do we conceptualize it and its role in forming moral selves? As anthropologists work to develop more theoretically rigorous understandings of morality and its place in ordinary life, new metanarratives and primal imaginaries have arisen. I have already proposed one—the "moral laboratory." Three alternative primal scenes, already hinted at in Chapter 2, offer vivid images that rely upon discursive pictures of moral becoming or that treat the ethical as a contrast space to the ordinary. Each has emerged primarily (though by no means exclusively) through Foucault's influence.

There is the image of an *artisan's workshop,* inspired especially by Foucault's formulation of the ethical project as "care of the self." Here we are introduced to an industrious space where artisans carefully, painstakingly fashion their crafts, following exacting aesthetic standards. What are they creating? What are their works of art? Themselves, as moral beings. And how are these selves made? Not through punitive measures exacted from a harsh judge or impartial assessments of an impersonal interrogator but, rather, the voluntary disciplining and monitoring of thoughts, acts, and especially bodies in line with the stylistic norms of the "guild" to which one has pledged oneself. The moral self is forged through a kind of apprenticeship in the "arts of existence" where the product of one's labor is nothing less than oneself. As Foucault puts it, the arts of existence are "those intentional and voluntary actions by which men not only set themselves rules of conduct, but also seek to transform themselves, to change themselves in their singular being, and to make their life into an *oeuvre* that carries certain aesthetic values and meets certain stylistic criteria" (1990b:10–11).

This spectacle of the artisan workshop emphasizes the connection between crafting the self and a pedagogical metanarrative. One trains in various disciplines to develop virtues proper to that particular craft guild—trains the body, the mind, and the soul. Social formations tend toward the hierarchical, novices laboring under the tutelage of masters. Authoritative texts and practices, often elaborately detailed, provide crucial guides for the telos that participants strive to attain. This aesthetic portrait foregrounds the day-to-day technologies of self-care that people draw upon to cultivate, or try to cultivate, virtuous characters. This is especially helpful when looking at the educational aspects of moral communities intended specifically for the cultivation of virtue and the moral transformation of self.[1]

An alternative, bleaker scenic cousin emphasizes the punitive characteristics of the everyday with its governmentalities and normalizing moral codes. The everyday emerges as a kind of *courtroom.* Fear prompts the cultivation of a moral self. Judith Butler gives an especially vivid rendering of this moral imaginary where we come to see ourselves as having an "I" with causal agency because we are blamed for the suffering of others. We are brought to trial, so to speak, and asked to justify our actions.[2] Through processes of interrogation our moral selves are born. Self-narratives are created as we—in terror—try to defend our own actions, casting a fearful look backward at our past deeds, giving ourselves a history.[3] When we are interpellated, that is, asked to recognize ourselves as the occupants of a particular subject position, this is not only a political act but also a moral one. We become who we are (as subjects) because we are accused of something and must defend ourselves. In this moral imaginary, like any accused person, we are required to give an account of our past (potentially "criminal") actions. This primal moral drama exposes the insidious work of power, power that is no mere imposition upon someone but—more horrifyingly—produces that someone in the first place. A someone further molded through ever-more refined technologies of discipline and punishment orchestrated through specific configurations of material space and institutionalized in neoliberal regimes.[4] Even when moral agency is wedded to practices of self-cultivation in the manner of the creative artisan, practical life easily reverts to a tacit enactment of repressive cultural norms in anthropological accounts.[5]

Yet a third type of social scene has been suggested. It is variously depicted as dynamic, disorderly, liminal, broken, transgressive, or Dionysian. Its wildness is characterized by its resistance to or life outside the moral ordinary. While differing in key respects, the works of anthropologists Zigon (2007, 2009) and Faubion (2011) illustrate this very nicely. Both demarcate a space for the "dynamic" or "breakdown" ethical moment in which the very norms and morals by which one ordinarily lives are themselves problematized and become objects of reflection, drawing inspiration from Foucault's discussion of "problematization" in their work. Such a scenic division makes it possible to preserve a special space for a kind of ethical self-creation that depends upon the suspension, however temporary, of the quotidian. In "limit experience" or breakdown moments, the very norms and morals by which one ordinarily lives are themselves disturbed. Through a scenic counter-juxtaposition, the ordinary serves as a negative counterweight, a kind of foil, to a potentially freer space of ethical reflection and transformation.[6] This imaginary of the disorderly is enormously useful for those who seek to introduce some notion of freedom and agency into their moral theories while at the same time continuing to emphasize the normative—even repressive—qualities of the moral ordinary.

The moral laboratory I describe is, by contrast to any of these, deeply buried within the everyday, and yet this is an everyday characterized not merely by the routine or the repressive but also by the new and unexpected. How does the moral laboratory stack up against these alternatives in illuminating the moral ordinary? To think about this, I turn to a central moral space, family life, and that most quotidian of activities, housekeeping.

CHORES

If there is one place that might seem the antithesis of the laboratory, especially a laboratory dedicated to the creation of new and unexpected experiences, the statistically improbable, it is the family's domestic sphere. Housekeeping chores do not intuitively appear the sort of activities in which Arendt's "miracles" of "the new" are likely to be born. The routines of upkeep, however necessary, seem rather to illustrate a cultural habitus of durable dispositions par excellence.

And indeed, this is the way that I initially heard them in countless accounts family members have given of their daily caretaking tasks. Mothers and grandmothers have been especially (to my mind inordinately) fond of reciting the little routines of family life. Not just in a single interview, but repeatedly, interview after interview. "Not again," I would groan to myself, upon hearing how daily skirmishes over bathroom times were negotiated, who had cell phone privileges, who had hidden the TV remote from his siblings, or where the best bargains for Cup-o-Noodles could be had. The topic of grocery store deals alone could take up an enormous amount of interview space. Efficiency and effectiveness seemed to dominate the logic of these stories. How can one feed nine people in the shortest amount of time? How can one pack in nutrients most easily for a child who has great difficulty eating? How can one share a bathroom among twelve people and get everyone out the door by 7:30 in the morning? This is the stuff of what Aristotle called *techné*, the kind of practical activity that involves skill, calculation about the best means to achieve given ends, and the mastery of skills—including social skills—to bring about a desired result.

The mystery for me was not that parenting kin would find it important to tell us, as researchers, about their daily routines or, given the extremely tight home economies that most of them lived with, their cleverness at finding inexpensive and easy-to-fix meals and snacks for their families. Rather, what I puzzled about was the sheer repetitiveness of these recitations and the frequency with which these served as answers to questions intended to elicit more emotional and less "fact-based" or detailed responses. "What has it been like for you to raise Nikolas?" we might ask. Or, "Has your life changed since your five grandchildren came to live with you?" Although we often asked concrete questions about home activities, we also asked questions like these, intended to direct people to reflective, big-picture descriptions. And still, from many parents or grandparents, these questions also elicited a concrete rehearsal of daily chores.

The emotional force of these litanies also surprised me. Routines were often recounted not as burdens or duties but with matter-of-fact delight and pride, even wonder at times, a sense of their dramatic import. Little family mysteries of "Who stole the remote?" as children squabbled over control of the television were recounted in cherished detail, with much wry laughter. I seemed to think I was hearing little stories or even lists devoid of plot, but people were clearly conveying something else, that these were significant events, tales that went to the heart of their lives. What was I missing?

To answer this, I introduce Delores, one such narrator of the puzzlingly mundane short story. I return to her family again and again throughout this book, though when I first met her, I didn't know how much she and her family would provoke my own rethinking. In this and the following chapter, I explore the making and remaking of ethical life as part of everyday family activities within Delores's extended household, where she served as matriarch along with two of her adult daughters and their children. In this chapter I discuss ordinary routines and chores as space in which virtues are cultivated.

I first met her in 1997 in the initial months of the study. She was in one of the waiting rooms of a large hospital where she brought her grandson, Leroy, for treatment of a congenital hip problem. Delores smiled in greeting, a round-faced grandmother with a mass of curly hair and a deep laugh. She introduced me to Leroy, a sturdy six-year-old whose smile was very like hers and who stayed shyly at her side. Many of my interviews with Delores were at her home. Delores lived in a part of Los Angeles area I had never been to, the town of Altadena, a community right next to old-money Pasadena. To get to her house, I drove by Pasadena's posh and stately homes until I crossed into the considerably less affluent streets where Altadena began. Delores lived in a pleasant, if bare, ranch-style house on a tree-lined street. Her neighborhood, although mostly poor, had a certain suburban graciousness. It also offered a startling wilderness backdrop, because Altadena butts up against the rugged San Gabriel Mountains. When the days are clear these craggy hills rear up starkly behind the town's streets. It seems as though, if you just keep driving up the sloping blocks, you will disappear into them.

Carolyn Rouse (another researcher on the team during the early years) and I did quite a lot of interviewing of Delores while sitting with our tape recorder at her front table next to the kitchen. She told us about Leroy and the rest of her family, recounting how she had found herself in a situation in which one of her daughters, Marcy, had lost custody of her five children. Delores was the only one in her extended family ready to take them in to live with her. She had to give up her career as a social worker, a job she liked, to help raise them. As she put it, stoically: "But I said [to myself], sometimes we just have to deal with situations. And we know we gotta put up with it no matter what. It's the rest of our lives. We gotta deal with it and adjust ourselves to dealing with it. I had to adjust myself . . . and adjust to these children."

She showed us around her house, the neighborhood, and the local school that several of her grandchildren attended. She was always ready to talk during these visits or when I met her at the hospital. And yet, I couldn't figure out for a very long time what she was trying to tell me. Here is a sample from an early interview in which she offers one of her many finely honed descriptions of her morning routines for organizing her five grandchildren to get off to school on time and her orchestration of snacks:

> So when I get them up—they take [their] bath at night—and then, when I get them up, then they, they always dress theyself. So, three years of me saying, "Hurry up, 'cos we wanna leave at 7:15, 7:20, taking you to school." And so that's not bad at all. And they, I make sure they, they get a snack—like chips and juice. And the other morning, they wanted peanut butter and jelly sandwich. So I allowed them to have peanut butter and jelly sandwich snack and juice. And so when they get home in the evening, they, they like Cup-o-Noodles. So every time I see them on sale—you can get the whole case for, like, for 3 dollars and something. Three dollars. Yeah. (She offers a satisfied smile.)

I only began to understand Delores when I could put these daily rituals of home care into a larger historical perspective, the perspective of a first person singular and plural, a family "we." It was in the context of unfolding family plots that small routines derived their dramatic import. I also began to see how much moral experimentation was involved in cultivating them. The matter-of-factness of Delores's statements belie the depth of the ethical currents attached not only to providing daily care for these children but her commitment to projects of moral transformation of the deepest sort, an embodiment of a project of narrative re-envisioning. She seemed to be telling us that the reimagining of oneself, one's family, one's life, is not a private introspective matter, some sort of internal story one tells oneself (though it may be that too), as much as an active, creative remaking of life through the development of new daily rounds of activities. In the local morality of the household, self-making and remaking are manifested most vividly, concretely, and compellingly in the creation and recreation of domestic routines.

In her repeated recitations of the procedures she establishes with the children, Delores reveals how the "adjustment" (as she put it) that came with quitting her job to care for her grandchildren is not a matter of technical virtuosity or even of stoical renunciation. It is a practice of love. Love shows itself as Delores describes her subtle reading of each child's little ways that she has incorporated into her wake-up system.

> Okay, Leroy when he don't get his way, he cries a lot. And what I do with Leroy, I hug him. It takes a lot of love, hugging with these children. And I tell Leroy, I say, "You growing up." He cries in the morning. My routine in the morning, getting childrens up for school, I hug them. I rub their back. And I say, "It's time to get up." Sometime Leroy get up crying. Don't want to get up. And so I have to sit there and pat him and hug him. I call him my big butterball. (She laughs.) And I say, "Come on, you my big butterball. Now come on, it's time to go." And so he'll get up and then he'll want to sit there and then he hug me. I say, "Give me big hug." And he'll hug me back and then he'll say, "Okay grandma, I'm going on and brush my teeth and get ready for school." I say, "That's a good boy." I get Candice up, and I have to hug, hug her, rub her back and say, "It's time to get up." I don't have much of a problem with Candice but Tina, it's a test to me every morning. Tina is a child, always like have a mind of her own. She wants to take her time. She wants to do it when she gets ready. So I don't [yell]. I hug her too. I have to hug her. And say, "Come on. You my big girl," or something like that. Say something sweet to her.

Delores continued in this manner until she had described her wake-up rituals with all five children.

Delores's family has had to learn to make and remake itself in the face of perils all too common to those who are poor and black. Rather than producing a durable habitus, home life is characterized by fragility. It is a precarious achievement and easily broken. In what follows, I examine a moment from their everyday life. This is a visit to the physical therapy clinic. At the time this occurred, part of routine care for Delores and her family involved regular visits for Leroy, whose hip condition made it difficult for him to walk or run. These visits were consequential because sometimes the treatment for this requires surgery. However, if treated early enough and if child and family are diligent enough in following a home exercise program for strengthening and stretching the legs, surgery can be avoided. When Delores received custody of Marcy's children, she began taking him to weekly physical therapy appointments and included the therapy exercises into family routines, as directed by the treating therapist. At the time of the session I describe, Leroy is six years old.

THE CLINICAL SESSION

Delores and Leroy sit together on chairs in one of the hospital's large rehabilitation treatment rooms. They wait for Patricia, the physical therapist, to arrive. Delores has brought some medical records with her. She also has a special notebook and a pen, prepared for notes. At a far corner of the room, opposite to Delores and Leroy, Marcy has placed her own chair. She only comes every once in a while to these sessions. She opens a large hardback book she has brought and begins to read, silently mouthing the words. No one speaks until Patricia arrives. Patricia, tall, blonde, quietly friendly, enters the room and speaks reassuringly to Delores and Leroy. She knows Leroy gets self-conscious in these sessions. No one pays attention to Marcy, who does not look up from her book. Leroy has weekly therapy sessions with his physical therapist. Delores *always* brings him, and she inevitably assumes the central maternal position, as she does in this session. The therapist directs her attention to Delores and Leroy. During their exchange, Marcy does not say anything and rarely looks up. Her face is grim, expression closed.

In the following exchange, Patricia is directing Leroy in exercises, and we can hear Delores repeating her instructions to Leroy, like a kind of assistant coach.

> *Patricia:* Now I want you to stand on your leg for as long as you can but don't count.
>
> *Dolores:* Now, don't count. Don't count.
>
> (Leroy stands on right leg but does not count.)
>
> *Patricia:* Good boy, good boy. Keep going. Okay, let's try the left one.
>
> (Leroy stands on left leg.)
>
> *Dolores:* Keep straight.
>
> *Patricia:* Now let's try to get to the door.
>
> (Everyone moves over to the door. Patricia backs Leroy up against the door.)
>
> *Patricia:* Okay, all the way against the door. Right in the middle.
>
> (Leroy lifts his right leg up while leaning against the door.)
>
> *Patricia:* Good. Keep it up. (She notices he is leaning against the door too much.) Aww you are cheating there, you are cheating. (Leroy changes position to satisfy the therapist.) Twenty! Good.

Having given him this small exercise, which also serves as a test of his strength, mobility, and endurance, the therapist turns to Delores to give her instructions about how to carry out exercises at home and what she should pay attention to.

> *Patricia:* Okay instead of having him do it without anything . . . stand him up against a door. And the longer he stands the better. You can use a chronological watch or with a second hand . . . something he can see. And the goal for him would be for him to stand on one leg for thirty seconds and then the next. The reason for that is that the longer he can stand on that leg the stronger he will be.
>
> *Dolores:* Okay, alright.
>
> *Patricia:* So this is really a good exercise. Just have him stand.
>
> *Dolores:* Okay.
>
> *Patricia:* If you try it you will see it is not easy.
>
> *Dolores:* Alright.

At session's conclusion, the therapist announces that she wants to review the exercises Delores has been doing with him at home. As Delores provides her a description, the therapist listens attentively and redirects her about a movement that Leroy should not be doing. She invokes the "doctor" (a higher authority) to underscore the seriousness of her statement.

> *Patricia:* Come sit right here. Sit. So which exercises are you doing?
>
> *Dolores:* Umm, the one that you just finished showing. And one with the leg stretch from the left to the right and the right to the left. We are doing that and to stand then on his side doing fifteen counts on the right and then the left. Then we have him stand like you just had him on one knee. Sometimes I have him face me and don't drop his shoulder just stand on the one leg. Until I count fifteen. And then I go from the right to the left and left to the right about three times with him. And then he will be throwing the ball with his brother and other friends. So they do exercises with the ball. And then he does the exercise with where he brings his knees all the way up to his shoulders. And umm, like jumping up and down on the . . .
>
> *Patricia:* He should not be doing that.
>
> *Dolores:* He should not be doing that?
>
> *Patricia:* Not yet.
>
> *Dolores:* He just did it for (pauses) uh, the first time I seen him do it was last night.
>
> *Patricia:* No jumping. That's what the doctor said.
>
> *Dolores:* Yeah, okay.

I have heard hundreds of conversations like this one in my years in rehabilitation clinics. Here again, as with housekeeping chores, it initially sounds much more like an example of routine *techné* than a moral matter. But, inspired by the scenes with which I opened the chapter, we can see how the moral enters this ordinary rehabilitation encounter.

Clinic as Artisan's Workshop

We could interpret this session as the fashioning of a kind of craft project. If Leroy is learning to discipline his body in certain ways, one might argue that he is (semi-) voluntarily involved in a process of self-mastery under the tutelage of an expert artisan (the physical therapist) who provides him the technologies necessary for his self-care. His grandmother serves as a lesser mentor, but one crucial to facilitating the transport of this craft technology from the clinic to home, where much of the work needs to take place. We can see this as *moral* work if we understand the technologies of self-care provided by experts as tools for the discipline not only of body but also of soul. He is training his soul, his very character, through moral arts of care that demand such things as willingness to endure moments of physical pain or tedium and willingness to refrain from forbidden pleasurable activities (e.g., "jumping").

Clinic as Courtroom

This exchange could be read, more perniciously, as a kind of trial. Grandmother and child are brought into a clinical courtroom where Leroy is caught cheating and Delores is found wanting in her supervision of Leroy's home program. Both are, if not punished, certainly tested, exposed, and corrected. The therapist exerts expert control, recruiting Delores not only to carry out a specified home program but also to extend her surveillance over Leroy. What Delores first announces as a kind of exercise, "jumping," turns out, as the therapist registers disapproval, to call for further defense by Delores, who then says (accounting for herself) that he has only done it once, just the night before in fact, and that she did not direct this activity but only happened to witness it. As in Butler's trial scene, Delores gives an account of herself that tries to proclaim her relative innocence. But still the therapist is not satisfied. She reiterates three times that this is not allowed, calling upon the authority of the doctor to underscore her reprimand.

But the interpretation I've given so far only hints at what Butler and Foucault (in his governmentality moments) mean us to pay attention to with this moral imaginary. To get at the way selves as subjects are pro-

duced through such exchanges, Butler and Foucault are directing attention not to interpersonal relationships but to structures of power. This
redirection to structures offers a more accurate reading of what is going
on between the therapist and Delores. Personally, this therapist quite
likes Delores. She finds her a cooperative and responsible caregiver and
enjoys working with her. But as an expert, drawing upon the discourses
and knowledge in which she has been trained, it is part of her job to
"try" Delores. Patricia's words and actions are bound up with very deep
and institutionally driven understandings of what constitutes responsible health care and the proper expert–client relationship.

What about Marcy, the mother who sits in the corner and doesn't
participate? This is where the "trial" imaginary helps expose how a subtle racism enters the picture and produces a stigmatized subject position.
Racism here depends upon these same authoritative discourses and
structurally defined roles. A good mother, according to the moral norms
governing appropriate clinic behavior, is certainly not one who sits on
the sidelines. The structure of rehabilitation depends upon the delivery of
massive amounts of "chronic homework" to patients and family caregivers who are expected to carry out home programs under the guidance of
health experts (Mattingly, Grøn, and Meinert 2011). When clients
(including family members) do not do their parts, they are labeled non-
compliant. This label can have extremely serious consequences. Children
can be taken out of their homes and put into foster care. This threat has
hung over many families who have been part of our study. The smallest
infractions can trigger the dreaded "home visit" by a social worker to see
whether he or she finds any evidence of parental neglect. Marcy's behavior presented a classic picture of negligence from a normative clinical
perspective. Although this did not bother Patricia, it annoyed many of
the therapists and aides who saw Marcy in the treatment rooms.

Their scathing dismissal of Marcy was brought home to us on the
research team with disconcerting clarity during an in-service presentation
of our research to the rehabilitation staff, which included occupational
and physical therapists and aides. In our presentation, to illustrate to the
hospital staff what we were studying, we chose to show a few minutes of
one of the videotapes of a treatment session with Delores, Leroy, and
Patricia. Because both Patricia and Delores felt they worked well together,
we thought it would be interesting to ask the staff what they thought was
effective about the interaction. Why were things going so well? How
would they analyze the ingredients of the encounter? The snippet of the
session we showed happened to be one where Marcy was sitting in the

background silently reading, as usual. But the staff were so incensed at Marcy's behavior that they paid no attention to our questions or to what was going on between Delores and Patricia at all. Instead, they directed all their attention to Marcy. "What an uninvolved parent!" they exclaimed indignantly. "She's not even watching! That's her *own* child and she doesn't lift a finger. She's letting her mother do all the work."

Their accusation bears upon a crucial indicator of an involved parent from a rehabilitation point of view. "Watching" is essential in this apprentice-like clinical encounter in which the parent is supposed to absorb cues about how to carry out the home physical therapy exercises. This includes paying attention to explicit instructions of the therapist and following commands but also following closely as the therapist directly treats the child to see how the exercises are correctly done. Although the staff never explicitly mentioned Marcy's race (a few of the aides were themselves African American), it is impossible not to see how Marcy is being "interpellated" in their comments. She is not seen as a bad mother in generic terms but in more specific race and class ones, as an irresponsible "ghetto mom."

Clinic as Moral Laboratory

The experimental qualities of this session are far less obvious. They concern Delores's effort to bring a family together. This is a family that includes not only the five grandchildren who now live with her, but, sporadically, Marcy. During these years, Delores was trying to do all she could to bring Marcy back to her children, to rescue her from the life she has been living. What the therapists who were so critical of Marcy completely missed was that this was no ordinary physical therapy—it was a trial run. The clinic served as a moral laboratory where Delores and her daughter Marcy were experimenting with motherhood itself. Marcy was struggling to transform herself, and in the most profound way, to become clean and sober after eighteen years—more than half her life—of being addicted to crack cocaine. The book she was reading during these therapy sessions was from Narcotics Anonymous. She was working on her twelve-step program, softly reading to herself. But could she do it? Could she become the kind of mother she wanted to be but was not? The odds were not in her favor.

One thing that Delores knew about her daughter was that she loved her children, although, Delores admitted, she could be "really mean" when she was high. But this, Delores felt, was not the real Marcy. "It was the drugs doing it," she remarked. "I think it was just the way that the drugs affect you." She added, "She used to be so hostile about things and I think the anger was from, she didn't like herself and she didn't like what she was doing to herself." During this early period of Marcy's sobriety, when Marcy accompanies her mother and son to the hospital, she provides evidence to herself and her mother of a possible new person she might become. This is not the person she is at that moment but a future self—the person she might be, a "real mother" to her children, one who is not mean, hostile, or angry, if only she can remain clean. She might not be ready to take the lead, to play the role that the therapists expect, but still, she is finding some way to participate in the routines of family life. Every such moment is a tryout in possibility, one that, in light of the statistics about drug addiction, was highly unlikely. She and her mother are pitting the possible against the probable.

As the analysis thus far shows, to reveal the deeply experimental qualities of little moments, it is necessary to recognize the temporality of these moments in which the *narrative* qualities of moral experiments become apparent as temporal moments and spaces in larger narrative trajectories. Laboratory moments like a clinic visit offer "beginnings" with all the fragility that Arendt counsels us to expect of action. They provide evidence of a sort, but is this evidence reliable? What Arendt highlights is that action spirals outward—it travels through social space and time, and often in unexpected directions. It is not surprising that the definition of experience as experiment is linked etymologically to another definition of experience—experience as a kind of journey, a passage. This second understanding of experience, as a passage—and a dangerous one—is a necessary counterpart. With the image of the perilous journey we are offered a narrative understanding of moral experience that is not about defending oneself after the fact or schooling oneself as an apprentice artist, but experiencing oneself to be living within possible narrative plotlines that stretch backward and forward in time, within a field of narrative potentiality.[7] In linking the narrative creation of a moral self to the idea of the "moral laboratory," I emphasize how small events can serve as experiments in possible futures, small inaugurations into something that might constitute a fleeting experience or might portend a future different than one had envisioned.[8]

THE PAST: LIFE ON THE STREET

Marcy's very presence at these clinical encounters represented one venture in an ongoing journey to leave "the street" and its ways, to find her way to a life as a mother. By her own account, she would never have been able to do this if Delores had given up on her. But Delores never did. Here is Delores, talking about her repeated attempts to rescue Marcy from the streets and bring her home:

> And there was times I would get up and I would go find her. Find some of her friends and I tell 'em "Don't lie to me. All I want to know is where is Marcy." And Marcy would see me and she'd say, "I'm getting ready to come." Maybe she was gone for a day or two. "I'm getting ready to come home Momma, I'm getting ready to come home." I said, "Yeah I know. You coming with me right now."

Delores recognizes that many people would have given up on their child, and overtly disapproved of what Marcy was doing. But for Delores, her judgment about rescuing her daughter represented the "best good" in this terrible situation. Delores remembered, "People yeah, people would tell me 'Oh you need to kick Marcy out. You ain't gonna never do this. She ain't never gonna never do nothing 'cause she know she can depend on you.'" But Delores disagreed. She felt it essential that Marcy knew she had a home she could come to. This was not some theoretical position but an expression of who she was, as a mother, of what her own capabilities were. As Delores put it:

> I've just never had a heart that I could just kick her out. I just not, couldn't do that. I don't know why. But, I didn't even, I don't think I even allowed myself to deal with the pain. I felt that she would be safer around me and when she wasn't around me and I didn't know where she was, that was the time only time I would worry. I would worry and pray. I said, "Lord send her home, wherever she is. Lord you know where she is. Send her home."

I offer the following account, a co-narrated story about the moment, after eighteen years, that Marcy finally comes home to her mother and her children. She is finally willing to go into a drug treatment program and leave the streets behind. Although I had heard various versions of this story before from Delores, this was the first time the two of them tell it together. The story was told about a year after Marcy had been clean. At this point, she and Delores had come to share many of the tasks of childrearing, a partnership that both looked upon with great pride. The story of the "final rescue" is told by Marcy and Delores a year after Marcy has gotten clean. They talk to two of us on the research team, Carolyn Rouse and me:

> *Delores:* A lot of the girls used to tell me, "Ooh, I wished we had a mother like you." Well, I just made up my mind, well, if I turn her to the street,

she gonna go worse. And if she knows she can come home and eat and sleep—and she'd come home—she would sleep three, four, or five days. (Marcy laughs.) She was walking and walking. So, one time—I really did. I got tired of it. I said, "I'm tired of this." I went and found her. And she didn't know I was coming. And all—

Marcy: But I was on my way home. (Marcy and Delores talk at the same time.)

Delores: I know it. I said—I know you was on your way home 'cause I'm coming down here to get you. And I told all her friends, "You better not lie. You better show me—tell me where she is." And they—I found her. She was getting something to eat. She said, "I was just getting ready to come home."

Marcy: (overlaps) I was gonna get on that bus. I was tired then. I was just going home (laughs). I was sad 'cause I had been gone, like, two whole weeks.

Carolyn: Do you remember the moment when you decided, "That's it"?

Marcy: Yup. I told my mom. I called to make me—put me on the waiting list. But the first program I called, I'm gone. I packed my bags, had them sitting by the front door.

Carolyn: What made you change your mind?

Marcy: As long as they was telling me to go to the program, I wasn't going. I ain't going till I got ready to go. That's why. I ain't going till I'm ready to go. When I get ready that's when I go. 'Cause if I go while y'all want me to go, it ain't gonna work.

Cheryl and Carolyn: Yeah. Yeah.

Marcy: It ain't gonna work.

Cheryl: Yeah.

Marcy: So when I got ready I got on three treatment programs.

Delores: We went to uh, Joe at the—they was doing an outpatient clinic for the city. . . . He said, "Marcy, you want to see some hard-core drug addicts?" He said, "Go down there."

Marcy: Right down on 5th Street, and that's where I went. I was standing around just watching them smoke right through it. I cried.

Delores: She said, "I cry every day, Momma. I cry every day. Look at these peoples."

Marcy: They sleep in cardboard boxes and all that stuff. You know, I ain't never had to do all that.

Cheryl: So, what do you think made you—what finally made you ready?

Marcy: Well, either you get tired . . .

Cheryl: Yeah.

Marcy: Or—you just get tired.

Although Marcy's ironic and pithy ending to this story makes leaving the street inevitable—you either "get tired" or you "get tired"—all of us in the room knew that those who have developed cocaine addictions in their teens, as Marcy had, were very unlikely to remain drug-free. You might "get tired," but can you actually quit?

AN UNCERTAIN FUTURE: THE DRILL TEAM AS MORAL LABORATORY

Will Marcy be able to maintain her sobriety against the odds? Even if she is able to do this, how will she find a way to inhabit this mothering role? Delores has many health problems. What will happen when Marcy must take over for her own mother, stepping in as a leader? Both Delores and Marcy worry about this. But Marcy continues to remain clean, and she begins to take on roles where she acts not simply as a follower of her mother or even as a partner but as a leader.

Most strikingly, her moral work of transformation takes her back to the street. Marcy decides to coach the local drill team and drum squad that several of her children are involved in (including Leroy, whose leg has gotten strong enough to allow him to play in the drum squad). She, too, was on a drill team as a young girl. She coaches a well-known local team in Altadena that performs competitively against teams all over the state. This new project of care allows her to reinhabit the streets in a very different way. Drill teams require great precision in choreographed movement and dance—there are endless hours of practice, and it takes great commitment to participate in them and coach them. The leaders of drill teams not only train but also develop their own choreography so that teams can present original work. Drill team and drum squad performances (a quintessentially African American art form that borrows from African dance movements, African American dance routines from earlier eras, and contemporary popular dance) perform in street parades that hundreds gather to watch, showing enthusiasm but also voicing critiques and comments if routines are not performed according to the highest standards. This is a very public space.

During these performances and parades, Marcy inevitably encounters many people she has known all her life, people who knew her as an addict and those who continue to use drugs. But as coach not only of her children but also of an important community program, she connects herself to the street as a participant of black pride and black history. In such events as the Pasadena Black History Parade, she helps to commemorate the black protest movements of the 1950s and 1960s, in this sense recalling yet another way to inhabit the streets. And yet, the experimental quality of such moments cannot be understated. Taking to the streets as a drill team leader is risky for Marcy, and it is not easy. She longs to leave the neighborhood and her past, to move her family elsewhere, away from the "mess," as she puts it. She stays for the sake of her mother, who is unwilling to leave the place she has long called home.

EVERYDAY EXPERIMENT VERSUS LIMIT EXPERIENCE: WHERE DOES THE ETHICAL LIVE?

The philosopher Stanley Cavell asks us to consider how the ordinary contains transcendent possibilities. There is a self-identity at least possible, Cavell claims, that is not simply ratified by our social roles and societally defined subject positions.[9] But transcendence or potentiality is not exactly a gift. If we are marked by moral potential, we are also poised for moral disappointment. Indeed, it is *disappointment* that deeply characterizes everyday life, he goes on to say, a "disappointment with the world as it is, as the scene of human activity and prospects" and an accompanying "desire for a reform or transfiguration of the world" (2004:2).

One might imagine that this disappointment would compel us to try to leave the everyday, or to find a better world in a place quite apart from the everyday. And of course, we can easily find this in many religious and philosophical practices. However, Cavell insists that this restless desire for "transfiguration of the world" also belongs to the quotidian. It is especially provoked by challenges associated with those personal relationships that matter most to us. He seems to suggest a kind of perverse longing that characterizes mundane life—it intimates possibility precisely as it disappoints. The existential paradox is that our moral projects do not simply allow us to realize our ideals, even if we might sometimes be able to achieve "an attainable next [moral] self" (2004:84). Undertaking these projects also presents us with an ongoing "task of accepting finitude" (2004:4).

Das offers an especially clear elaboration of the everyday from a Cavellian perspective that reveals its distance from the more usual ways in which anthropologists have envisioned it. She states, "Everyday life can be understood in many ways. Everyday life might, for instance, be thought of as the site of routine and habit, within which strategic contests for culturally approved goods such as honor or prestige take place.

For others, everyday life provides the site through which the projects of state power or given scripts of normativity can be resisted." But, Das argues, our attachment to routines and habits is inflected by another affect: "The experience of the everyday [is] also the site of trance, illusion and danger" (2007; 2010:376). That the ordinary is *also* a space of illusion and danger is of paramount importance to a Cavellian understanding of moral striving. It means that "to secure the everyday, far from being something we take for granted, might be thought of as an achievement" (Das 2007; 2010:376).

I add that everyday routines are not only achievements in the face of a backdrop of crisis and trauma but also because they intimate possibilities for transcendence. They feed an ongoing practical and dogged hope to create something morally better. The attempt by Delores and Marcy to enact a ground project of mothering in the face of Marcy's addiction is nothing if not chancy. Success is always against the odds. As Delores and Marcy demonstrate, everyday rituals and routines not only demand planning, learning, and reinvention as new situations arise, they embody the qualities of a precarious enterprise in which the everyday is not so much transgressed as taken up in new ways. Natality here is not a matter of moving dramatically outside ordinary life demands and routines as the notion of "limit experience" suggests. Nor does the idea of a moral breakdown of an unreflective everyday habituation adequately capture what is going on in their lives. It is more accurate to say that their ground projects of life engagement demand a kind of transcendence of what already exists. Their "moral striving" does not leave behind but rather depends upon the cultural resources of the everyday to try to bring something new into existence. Through the loving and vigilant creation of routines of care, home figures as a sanctuary, but a sanctuary that cannot be relied upon.

Their situation also reveals one way that critique of subject positions may be embedded in ordinary life. In the efforts of Marcy and Delores to create a new family life, the category of the Superstrong Black Mother is also indirectly questioned. It becomes morally problematic because it cannot simply be inhabited. Delores may epitomize its virtues, but she resists a normative gaze that would preclude Marcy from coming to take up this position. Delores takes the lead in experimenting—against the odds—within all sorts of everyday spaces in her efforts to create a mothering team with her daughter. In doing so, she challenges received wisdom about long-term addicts, a normative view promoted by some members of her community (friends, other family members) who chastise her, saying she should just "give up" on her daughter after so many years. Together, Delores and Marcy build a whole repertoire of experiences that give evidence to support their improbable hope. Marcy counters her skeptics every time she takes to the streets of her old neighborhood as, for example, a drill team leader striving to participate in street life in a new way, as a good mother.

Without offering a complex moral portrait of the everyday, one gets the sense that in ordinary life, moral technologies are already firmly in place, and this misses the many ways people experiment with, critique, and modify the very traditions they have inherited or in which they have "schooled" themselves as part of their self-making projects.[10] Thus, I do not demarcate a special realm of "ethical freedom" that is distinct from the moral ordinary. Instead, I highlight aspects of everyday action and practical reasoning that point toward its transcendent possibilities and its disappointments. I'm not contesting that certain kinds of breakdown moments (and I offer some in the following chapter) can intensify reflection and critique of moral norms. But the concomitant implication that the ordinary is devoid of these qualities is costly, because it disguises the resources for moral experimentation, critique, and transformation that are ongoing potentialities within everyday social practices.

Small moments like a clinic visit and a drill team performance can represent something enormous. These activities speak to a cherished *ordinariness,* to the cultivation of "significant routines" (Grøn 2005; see also Lawlor 2003, 2012). Families like Delores's are frequently gripped by personal and family dramas that are of consuming interest to those involved. Turbulence, uncertainty, and drama are such pervasive qualities that ordinary routines are not the daily expression of a habitual way of life culturally inherited so much as a fragile achievement, a hard-won moment of mundaneness. Under such circumstances, the ordinary is freighted with a special moral weight, and it can acquire an unexpected symbolic density.

CHAPTER 4

Luck, Friendship, and the Narrative Self

Moral change and moral achievement are slow; we are not free in the sense of being able suddenly to alter ourselves since we cannot suddenly alter what we can see and ergo what we desire and are compelled by.

—Iris Murdoch (1970:39)

Western antiquity offered a view of the human condition that was not self-sustaining. In this cosmology, not only were humans subordinate to the gods, the gods who ruled them were fickle and could not be trusted. Through no fault of their own, humans could be subjected to bad luck because of celestial recklessness, malice, or sheer godly indifference to human concerns. This was a matter of considerable worry and debate among ancient philosophers. How did one create a good life when life was, at best, under partial control? When fate played such a significant role in shaping human destiny? Contemporary moral philosophers calling upon the ethics of antiquity consider additional sources of luck and its volatile effects on human lives.

What follows is a story about bad luck.

THE KITCHEN ACCIDENT

Two years after Leroy's clinic visit that I described in the previous chapter, one of the children in Delores's household, a very young boy named Willy, was badly burned and had to be rushed to the hospital. This event was the outcome of an unfortunate and unintentional configuration of actions, each of them small in and of themselves. At the time of the accident, Delores's extended household included not only Marcy and her five children, but also Delores's youngest daughter Sasha and her son Willy. During this period in the family's life several good things had happened. Marcy had been drug-free for nearly three years. The family had established a relatively smooth domestic routine among Delores and her two daughters who shared child care tasks. Leroy no longer needed physical therapy; he had nearly full use and range of his body. He continued in the drum squad that accompanied the drill team Marcy coached, one where several of his sisters also participated. He lost some of his earlier pudginess, now getting regular exercise in marching practices. It was clear that he was never going to be a football player like his older brother Ralph, who was a quarterback for the local high school team (to the family's joy), but his drumming folded him into the family in another way. This shared activity was a big hit among the children. We sometimes videotaped the parades in which they performed and brought the DVDs to show them. They would laughingly pile onto Delores's large bed. (Her bedroom had a television and served as a family center.) They watched intently, asking us to replay them again and again, pausing the recording to look more carefully when one of them came into view, admiring their uniforms, poking gleeful fun at one another's lapses in perfect routine.

And then one day Willy, just a year and a half old at the time, toddled into the kitchen after his nine-year-old cousin Shareen, who had decided to fry some bacon. She wasn't an experienced cook and did not realize that bacon required no grease. She heated oil in the frying pan and dropped the bacon in. It immediately splattered uncontrollably, and in trying to figure out what to do, she did not notice that Willy had somehow managed to reach up to the stove. He tipped the frying pan on his head, covering the lower part of his face with burning oil. Delores heard the screams and immediately called 911 for an ambulance. Sasha was not at home. She had left the house a few minutes earlier to pick up her cousin. It was a short trip—she would be back in twenty minutes so she didn't worry about leaving her son in the care of her mother, her sister, and Willy's older cousins. There were plenty of people around and Shareen had promised to look out for him. By the time Sasha returned from her errand, a few minutes later, Delores and Willy and Shareen were already in an ambulance on the way to the hospital.

LUCK AND THE FRAGILITY OF ACTION

New projects of becoming may be set in motion through the accidents of fortune. So, a chain of events—Sasha's quick trip to pick up her cousin, her inexperienced niece's decision to fry some bacon, her son's unexpected ability to pull himself up high enough to tip over a frying pan—these conspire to provide radically altered circumstances and set a new story in motion. Such events not only expose inadequacies that were once unnoticed, they demand virtues not needed before. Accidents create new situations that demand new or more well-developed virtues in order to even perceive a "best good" in uncharted waters.

For Delores's family, this traumatic event created an immense rupture. Through Delores's many efforts, theirs had become a close-knit multigenerational household, even if fractious at times. Squabbles and rifts would periodically arise not only among the children but also between Sasha and Marcy. However, Delores's presence was so powerfully felt and her daughters were so loyal to her that they tried to work out their differences. But now, one of Marcy's children had not watched out for Willy, and Sasha felt betrayed. "I lost my trust," Sasha said. She found herself bitter and angry. In addition, Sasha was confronted with a new, unfamiliar maternal task—how to care for a child who now had many medical needs and whose face had become disfigured, perhaps permanently so. This demanded the acquisition not only of technical skills (how to dress a wound, how to entice her son to wear the medical face masks he hated), but a project of moral becoming—how to gain the strength (as she often put it) to become a good mother to this child under these circumstances. Delores played a crucial role in guiding Sasha in both these tasks.

Perhaps no one is as eloquent about the capriciousness of the social and the fragility of action as Hannah Arendt, and so I return to her again. Action is frail most of all, she tells us, because we are simply unable to accomplish anything properly called action by ourselves. It is "never possible in isolation" but needs the "surrounding presence of others" (1958:188). Action necessarily occurs in "constant contact with the web of acts and words of other men" (1958:188). Because we must enlist the cooperation of others, we are vulnerable to them. Examining Greek and Latin terms for the verb "to act," Arendt notes that it has two parts, a beginning (which a single person can do), and an achievement— seeing the enterprise through, which is necessarily a social, cooperative accomplishment. Other actors in the scene commit consequent deeds. They take up the story that has been started and move it along in potentially unexpected and even unintended directions. Action and suffering are like two sides of the same coin, she argues, because the stories an actor tries to set in motion may not be those that actually unfold.

Furthermore, actions are boundless because possible consequences are endless. Actions "act in a medium where every reaction becomes a chain reaction and where every process is the cause of new processes. Since action acts upon beings who are capable of their own actions, reaction, apart from being a response, is always a new action that strikes out on its own and affects others" (Arendt 1958:190). This open quality of action cannot be contained within any laws or institutions. Arendt continues, "The smallest act in the most limited circumstances bears the seed of the same boundlessness, because one deed, and sometimes one word, suffices to change every constellation" (1958:190). Arendt counsels that we are no longer aware of this vulnerability of action because history has forgotten it, gradually developing a vision of social life divided between rulers (who begin) and followers (who execute according to orders) (1958:189). (Or, in a long tradition of social theory, a bifurcation in which the rulers are no longer persons at all but rather the social structures or systems themselves.[1])

MORAL BECOMING AND THE NARRATIVE SELF

I do not address how or why "bad luck" happens, but rather, what kinds of moral tasks does it set? This chapter explores the relationship between something like "luck" and the project of moral becoming, scrutinizing the cultural resources that mundane routines and material spaces provide for this effortful moral task. I have proposed that first person virtue ethics demands a complex narrative portrait of the self. Moral decisions emerge as aspects of unfolding narrative histories, including biographical ones. I follow virtue ethicists who reject the picture of a moral agent "thin as a needle" in Iris Murdoch's wondrously dismissive prose, an agent who "appears in the quick flash of the choosing will" (1970:53). Murdoch insists that it is better to think of moral agency as a painstaking process demanding "discernment and exploration," which is, as she says, a "slow business." The slowness is related to a key feature of moral transformation—it requires a change in perception itself, a re-envisioning of the situations one faces and of oneself. But perception, so integral to moral action, is very difficult to shift even when one "wills" to do so. Murdoch offers the hypothetical example of a woman who simply cannot abide her new daughter-in-law. Everything this young woman does annoys her. Her looks, her manner of speech, her tone of voice, the way she walks—all are irritating. And yet, this mother loves her son and her son loves this young woman. She is unhappy with her annoyance, believes it petty. But it is not a matter of simply willing herself to perceive her daughter-in-law differently in some moment of choice. Rather, she has to work at it painstakingly, retraining her perception, learning to see the charm in what she earlier experienced as abrasive. "Love," Toni Morrison wrote, "is not a gift. It is a diploma." But it is a strange kind of diploma for this is a peculiar kind of school. "How do you know when you graduate?" she asks. "You don't. What you do know is that you are human and therefore educable and therefore capable of learning how to learn. . . ." (1997:141)

Murdoch defines this kind of effort as *moral reorientation*. Such reorienting involves "the acquiring of new objects of attention and thus of new energies as a result of refocusing. The metaphor of orientation may indeed also cover moments when recognizable 'efforts of will' are made, but explicit efforts of will are only a part of the whole situation" (Murdoch 1970:56). Murdoch emphasizes the internal efforts this kind of moral re-envisioning entails. I pay attention to the play between this internal work and something more external, more intersubjective—the world of social action. My characterization has resonance with phenomenological anthropology's studies of moral transformation, especially Csordas's (1994) influential discussion of religious practices that involve the cultivation of certain "somatic modes of attention."[2]

SASHA'S PROJECT OF MORAL TRANSFORMATION

Sasha portrays her most difficult struggle as battling her initial bitterness and anger. It was difficult for Sasha not to be angry at Shareen, but she knew that her niece was not only "really, really sorry" but also felt horribly guilty. "She couldn't even, when I got to the hospital, she couldn't even look at me," Sasha reported. In the hospital Sasha acts generously—she hugs her niece. But this generous act is only a moment in an ongoing effort not to become bitter or blame anyone for what happened. This internal effort is at the heart of Sasha's many stories about caring for her child. Here is one of many quotes on the matter:

> It was, oh God, so, so painful for me . . . 'cause you first, I mean, you want to be mad. That's what I wanted to be initially. I wanted to be mad.

She has labored to combat this. "I tried really hard not to be angry, not to be bitter, because I know how it can make a person. . . . ." It becomes Sasha's task to cultivate just those sorts of virtues that will enable her to relinquish her position as critical judge of Shareen. Much greater compassion is needed than she originally possesses. She is grateful that despite her anger, the feeling of hurt is what predominated. And even her hurt has gradually subsided. She has been able to move on, even to consider herself lucky for her child who has survived his surgeries and is "so, so smart." She couches this moral reorientation in the language of healing. As she puts it, "I healed from my hurt."

One of the most significant contexts Sasha draws upon to make decisions about how to care for Willy, or to envision what kinds of moral decisions she faces, is her own unfolding life. She recalls how unfamiliar the world was in which she was suddenly plunged. This new world has confronted her again and again with new moral challenges. Sasha states:

> No matter how you think you've conquered it, in one way, you know it's always something new that comes up. When you think, "Okay, I've got this down," you know, something new happens. Maybe there is a new surgery the physicians tell you about, and you have to face your fears all over again, or maybe he will be teased now that he's in school, and you'll have to deal with that.

Issues that demand definite decisions, like whether to proceed with a surgery or not, are faced by Sasha gradually through both discussion with friends and family, heartfelt self-reflection and active thought experiments about what the possible consequences of her decisions might be. She describes in detail the agony she faced in agreeing that her son should have his initial surgery, a horror that never completely diminished as he underwent subsequent surgeries:

> They [clinicians] told me all the bad things that could possibly happen. Like he could lose consciousness and die. You know, because we're paralyzing his body from the neck down with medicines. . . . They tell me that . . . his throat could swell while in surgery and cause him to lose his breath.

These are moral decisions and not merely practical ones because they demand that Sasha herself change, become a different kind of mother, in order to be able to choose the best good for her son. In her case, she has to battle a kind of paralysis that sweeps over her when she considers what could happen to her son during surgery. Already she was still "dealing with the idea that he got burned," which was no small trauma, but then she is required to "deal with the fact that they might come out of this room and tell me that my son died." Deciding to allow her son to undergo a series of surgeries to repair the scars on his face must be done from a place of strength; each one terrifies Sasha. She presents the problem of making the right decision not as a matter of willing something, of making a choice at a particular moment, as much as taking on the larger task of how to be the kind of person capable of facing such tough choices, acting from a position where she has the moral strength to perceive and act on the best good. It is the cultivation of a particular way of being a mother for her son that she sees as her biggest task. She remarked once, plaintively:

> Everyone would say you have to be strong for [Willy]. But, I mean, how do you, be strong, you know? It's like, that's like, that's my kid. . . . I'm vulnerable, you know what I mean? Because this is my kid and he has just suffered, you know, something I never imagined.

In order to choose whether or not to proceed with surgery from a place of strength, she must face her own vulnerability. These situations that must be "dealt with" are not isolated decision points but events in an emergent and uncertain life story. She situates the ongoing work of making good choices about how to care for Willy within a broader project of remaking her life, including reorienting her own moral perspective. She believes this horrible accident has caused her to develop a finer moral sensibility. She has had to confront her own callousness toward those with disabilities or disfigurements. Willy's misfortune

> made me a better person. . . . 'Cause I used to be like really judgmental. Like, "Oh, what's their problem?" Or, you know, "What's wrong with them?" But it kind of made me realize that, you know, people do the same thing that I did to others. You know, to my son."

She has been forced to become more sensitive to the pernicious effects of physical stigma. She has also been confronted by the limitations of the care she can provide. Even as she tries to shield her son from the derision of others, she knows this is impossible.

> And I try to protect him from that, you know. And I know no matter how I try to protect him that there's gonna be someone out there that's gonna be like "Ohh. You know or some kid out there's gonna be like, "You're ugly," or something like that. But he takes it in stride, he takes it in stride. And I'm really proud of him, you know? And that's that.

Her moral re-envisioning has allowed her to embrace the pain of others—to quite literally *see* others, those with disabilities and disfigurements, differently. She even finds moments of gratitude. "Dealing with Willy in hospitals, she once remarked, "I've seen so many people that have been burned. He had this one little boy that was in the hospital with him. He was probably like one year old, like Willy. He got burned with acid. You know, he lost his ear, he lost an arm. It made me appreciate my son's burns. It made me really, really appreciate them because he was burned bad, but he could have been burned worse." This moral growth is only part of her changing life story, however. Her journey is as much about loss as it is a pilgrim's progress. Sasha reluctantly admits it has involved not only immediate sacrifice but the likely long-term surrender of a cherished and constitutive ground project.

Sasha is a dancer. When she describes her dancing her whole face lights up, her small body poised for movement. She has been trying to save money to move to New York. There is a good dance program at New York University that she has heard about and she wonders whether she might be able to get in. Perhaps she might even be able to start her own dance company or open a dance studio someday. At the time of Willy's accident, she was dancing with a troupe that frequently performed to enthusiastic audiences. She was building a local reputation. Remembering this period a few years later she commented, "My life was going well. It was on a good path. It was, I was doing what I loved to do. I had my son and I was dancing and you know, life was pretty great."

When the accident happened, this part of her life came to an abrupt halt. She refused to leave Willy's side:

> And then, he got burned. And it altered my life in a great way. In a major way. I wasn't able to do the things that I had been because he needed twenty-four-hour care. And I didn't want to put that burden on my mom, you know, or, any other one.

Sasha's entire orientation to her life is radically altered, subjected to a new kind of review—what Taylor would describe as "strong evaluation," that is, evaluation in terms of one's assessment of the highest goods. As Sasha put it:

> It just really made me re-evaluate life itself. You know, and how valuable life is. Because in that instant, I mean, he was one years old. He could have died, you know, the burns could have been so severe where he didn't make it.

Sasha's reorientation is not a solo task. It involves many social practices and is aided by family and friends. Every time Willy has gone in for a surgery—and especially during the first surgery when he had a thirty-day hospital stay—his family and Sasha's friends from church kept him company, crowding noisily into the hospital room, to the annoyance of the nursing staff. These actions and the messages that Sasha received about how she should respond to her son's injury have helped her in relinquishing her anger. No one told her to "be mad," she remembers. Instead, "I had positive people around me the whole time," and they counseled her to "just think good thoughts and . . . what you think is what will happen."

The "we-ness" of her accounts underscore how the whole family has been faced with the moral task of reorientation, a "we" framing echoed by Marcy and Delores who also experienced this as a dramatic family event. At first, Sasha says, this horrifying incident "crippled" the family: "When Willy got burned, it crippled us." But then things changed. The family "embraced" Willy and the pain of what happened; in fact, as the three mothers in this family have often said, this tragedy brought them together in a new way. They responded to it by learning to become stronger. All the children became involved with Willy's care. Everyone wanted to bathe him, to clean his wounds. In the initial days when he came home from the hospital, Willy was the central figure in the household. Sasha remembers:

> It was like everybody needed a role to be able to function. You know, like everybody wanted to either bathe him or to clean his wounds or you know have something to do with him directly. You know for everyone to feel like okay, I'm a part of this, you know. Or, I'm dealing with this, you know?

In Sasha's mind, this radically transformed family life, knitting them together as never before. She described it in this way:

> As a family, we've never embraced anything, so when he got burned it just like, everybody just grabbed it and hugged it and was like "This belongs to me." You know, even though it was like really hard and painful for all of us, but it, we had to deal with it as a family versus just me dealing with it as mom, or my mom dealing with it as grandmother. We just took it and dealt with it.

Small actions, such as the cousins' insistence on helping to take care of Willy, take their (moral) meaning as episodes in this unfolding family story.

When Willy was first hurt, Sasha turned for moral assistance to an admired and particularly close cousin, a "super-Christian," as Sasha described her, who

> just talked to me about Jesus, and how God was gonna take care of it. . . . I just have to believe that it's gonna be okay, you know? Then, and then after that, that's when the process of healing will begin.

But the process of moral change and family re-envisioning is most intimately bound up with the gradual reshaping of home routines. Sasha stresses that family healing occurred through actions. She once noted that in her family it is through such practices of care, rather than talking together or focusing on emotions, that people tried to heal their collective hurt.

> Because, I mean we honestly, we've never sat down as a family and really talked about it. We just embraced it, and moved from there. We never really sat down. Well I've never sat down with them, you know. And none of them have ever come to talk to me about it. Like well let's sit down and talk about the situation. Like okay, "This, this hurt." "This really affected me." Or "This is how I felt." We never did like that. We never did that. But everybody grabbed it and just made it a part of them.

But this does not happen as smoothly as Sasha intimates here. There was no immediate pulling together. Instead, this only happened after some failed experiments on her part. Although Sasha continued to live in the extended family household, she initially experimented with new modes of protection. She isolated herself and Willy from everyone else, hovering over him continually, not only keeping him inside the house but trying to keep other family members away from him. "My trust then with leaving my son with people, I couldn't do it for a long time. . . ." For several years, Sasha continued to worry about whether or not she could leave her son at home alone. She said, "I wonder sometimes, is it or isn't it safe to leave him? If I leave him this time what will happen this time?" She was even warier of allowing him to play with children outside the home or to go to school. "And I wouldn't put him in school for a long time because of his scars and stuff," she admitted. "I tried to protect him, you know, from other kids, from people."

When Willy first came home from the hospital, Sasha also tried to find ways to deal with the stigma of his disfigurement. Her initial strategy was to remake home itself. She covered every mirror in the house so that Willy, one and a half at the time, couldn't see his face. "I wouldn't let him see himself," she said. This undertaking was not successful, however, because it was not supported by other family members, most notably Delores. In the remainder of this chapter, I explore Delores's crucial role in Sasha's life as a moral mentor, someone that the philosopher Cavell (in some ways following Aristotle) would describe as a friend.

FRIENDSHIP AND THE MORAL SELF

She is a friend of my mind. She gather me, man. The pieces I am, she gather them and give them back to me in all the right order.

—Toni Morrison, *Beloved* (1987:520)

Virtue ethicists inspired by Aristotle tend to have a lot to say about friendship, one of the key goods he deemed essential for moral flourishing. The moral vocabulary surrounding friendship in the context of family life, particularly as developed by Cavell, provides an immensely illuminating window in which to explore the social dimensions of care and its demands for moral transformation that Sasha faces. I use Cavell to think with because he explores moral transformation as an intimate interpersonal task, one that requires the assistance of significant others with whom one has a serious a committed bond. In the previous chapter, I drew upon Cavell to portray everyday life as characterized by its transcendent potentialities. Friendship is necessary for realizing these potentialities, Cavell insists. Transformative work takes self-reflection and self-critique, and friends provide an essential resource for this.

In Cavell's ethics, one is confronted not by an impartial judge (a sort of third person arbitrator) who demands justifications for one's actions. Rather, one encounters oneself and one's way of life in a questioning way through *conversation* with friends. Conversation, Cavell remarks, plays the same role as calculation in utilitarian schemes and moral law in Kantian ones. In conversation (obviously, conversation of a particular sort), one is confronted by a particular personally significant other—a friend, in fact—who is essential for reflective self-consideration. But there is another difference operating here too. Although in utilitarian and Kantian schemes, I am required to justify myself "to offer or refuse reasons on which I am acting" (2004:49), in these conversations with friends, something else is required. I am asked to "reveal myself" to an intimate other, and through this revelation, my response is *not* justification in front of an impartial judge (as in these alternative moral frameworks) but something fundamentally dialogical. Cavell describes this as "one soul's examination of another" (2004:49).

Thus, self-questioning depends upon the presence of another person who has some moral standing with me. It relies on a first person moral perspective, in other words. Although in third person moral schemes, someone's personal relationship with me is of no consequence, this is not true here. If you confront me, there is no universal moral imperative that can carry the argument or compel me to listen, Cavell argues. Rather, "You had better have some standing with me from which you confront my life, from which my life matters to you, and matters to me that it matters to you" (2004:50). I listen to the advice of my friend because I believe that this friend is someone to be respected. More than this, I heed the advice, or at least find myself compelled to be confronted by it, because it comes from a person who knows and cares about me. The being known and cared for is an essential part of what gives that person moral standing.

We can see that Delores has played such a role with Sasha, putting persistent pressure on Sasha to re-enter everyday family life and to allow the other children in the family to help care for Willy. Delores was the one who challenged Sasha's approach to safeguarding Willy by preventing him from seeing his disfigured face. Delores was adamantly against her actions. Sasha reported their conversation:

> My mom said, "You can't do that to him." She said "Because you're forcing him into a place that he's not ready to go." And so, I didn't understand it. I was just like, "What are you talking about?"

Although Sasha did not initially accept Delores's position, she subsequently came to understand it, as she discloses in a later interview.

> And when she, when she brought it to my attention, that's when I began to deal with it. And then once I dealt with it, it was just like, "I don't care what anyone thinks." I just reassure my son, you know. "Don't let anybody tell you different. You know, you're not different from anybody else."

What is especially striking about this reported ongoing conversation between Delores and Sasha is that that what Delores "brought to [Sasha's] attention" is not that she shouldn't cover the mirrors but something much more profound. Sasha comes to understand that it was she, and not her son, who couldn't "deal with" his disfigurement. Delores serves the crucial role of friend by pointing not to a simple error in moral judgment but a whole way of understanding how to support one's child who is going to be confronted by social stigma. Hiding is not the answer; coming to accept one's physical imperfections is. But this means challenging the way the world is likely to see you, developing an internal resilience that can withstand the scorn of others. If Sasha wants her son to think that he is not different from, or less than, others, she must herself come to see her child in this way. She must summon a new kind of moral courage she has not needed before, the kind that will allow her to not "care what anyone thinks" about her son's scars.

When Cavell insists that moral transformation is not merely an internal process but an interpersonal one, the examples he chooses to illustrate his claims are taken from a genre of Hollywood remarriage comedies of the 1930s. These sparklingly written films showcase fast-paced, clever dialogues among the key protagonists. They are, quite literally, conversational. In drawing upon his idea of conversation I extend this notion to include a less sparkling, indeed less verbal form of dialogue, one that is rooted in household chores, the activities that constitute the daily rounds of care. In the thirteen years I knew this family before Delores's death, she was at the helm in keeping the household together, and her primary avenue of action was the crafting and recrafting home routines in response to the changing circumstances of their lives together. When Willy was hurt, Delores did not so much converse with Sasha as steer her and the whole family toward new ways of being together in which care for Willy became a family project.

Family routines may offer the material ground for reimagining Willy's new identity, but in what way? What kind of "special child" is he? The willingness of others to care for him gives him a special moral role in the household, as a kind of "healer." Sasha also emphasizes how smart he is. She is quick to provide evidence. "Look how he knows his colors!" "Look how well he reads!" she exclaims as he grows older. Gathering such evidence is crucial not only to counter the stigma of physical disfigurement, but to refute the clinical warning that he might suffer learning delays because his mouth was so burned he couldn't speak for two months.

> They told me his mouth got burned shut, and so he couldn't speak for like two months. They said that it, it would register to his brain. That, you know, so he might have a disability with learning. And he doesn't have that. They told me that his eye, you know, all, all these things could possibly go wrong with his eye, you know. And none of the things has happened. Call it fate. You know, he's a miracle. I strongly believe in God. I just think that he's destined to be someone great.

Sasha can tell very difficult stories that expose her own flaws or the flaws of those she loves. When it comes to Willy, though, she is unwavering in her proud accounts in which he is not only unbothered by his scars but is a heroic moral rescuer and teacher of herself and her family. Delores offers another view, which she steadily introduces into family life. She has many strategies for countering Sasha and for operating as a Cavellian friend. Delores wants Sasha to appreciate how ordinary her son is. We can see this with particular clarity in a story Delores instigated that became part of family lore.

THE "DOG FOOD DINNER": THE CULTURAL SHAPE OF THE MORAL ORDINARY

Delores created many small moments within the routines of everyday family life to signal that Willy, however his face may be changed, is neither victim nor hero. He is still a headstrong child who can make any-one laugh. She told many stories to reinforce this. Here is one in which cooking for the children becomes a chance to craft a story in which Willy's agentive, witty, and cantankerous qualities are revealed. The household routine in this family is that on days when Delores cooks dinner, she "likes to start it early," and then people can eat whenever they please. She laughingly recounts how Willy asked for his food and what he thought about her cooking.

She tells this story to a group of other parents and members of our research team. This was during one of our Collective Narrative Group meetings, which Mary Lawlor and I have co-run for fifteen years as part of our longitudinal ethnographic study. During the primary years of the study (1997–2011), we held between two and four such meetings each year. During the meetings families talked about their experiences of car-ing for their children with one another and the research team. (Since the research officially ended in the spring of 2011, we have met just once a year for a "family reunion.") Delores was a regular member, and the other families already knew her, as well as Sasha. They had heard humorous stories about Willy before, almost always recounted by Delores. In the dog food narrative, Delores offers a glimpse of a young child who is far from a victim, a healer or a hero. Not only can he be safely cared for when Sasha is away from home, her story illustrates, he exhibits the ability to take good care of himself. She pulls in Sasha (also present in the group) as co-narrator. It is important that Delores does not simply help to create the experience she later recounts, but that putting this experience into a narrative, and telling and retelling that narrative—charging Sasha to be a co-narrator—is her means of memo-rializing such moments.

> *Delores:* I like to start my dinner early, and so Willy came to me and said last night, he said, "I'm ready to eat." And I said, "Okay, I'm gonna fix your plate right now." And he always says something funny. Last night I had barbeque chicken and cabbage. And he says, "This is dog food." (Group laughs.) And I said, "What did you say?" "This is dog food!" And I said, "Well don't eat the cabbage, eat the meat." And he tastes the meat and says, "That is pretty good." Later in the evening he comes back for more food. About ten o'clock last night he came back. He said, "I'm ready to eat again." And I said, "Remember you told me I cooked dog food?" He laughs and I tell him, "Eat the cabbage." And he ate the cabbage. He said, "This is pretty good, this is pretty good." And he ate it all. And so when Sasha got home I said, "Sasha, your son said I cooked dog food!" (Dolores laughs.) And [Sasha] asked him, "What did you say?" (She turns to Sasha.)

> *Sasha:* (reluctantly joins in at her mother's solicitation) He told me he ate dog food. (Group laughs.)
>
> *Dolores:* I said, "Out of all the years I've been cooking I never cooked dog food for nobody."

This joking episode is further elaborated by Willy's cousins. They went to the store and brought back some dog food that they then presented to Delores. Delores adds this epilogue to the co-narrative amid much laughter by the rest of us. Although Sasha consistently identifies her son as a gifted boy and a family healer who is somehow above the fray, Delores actively creates a different child, one who is "ordinary," the kind of boy willing to insult his own revered grandmother. Delores's comic rendition furthers another kind of family identity attached to Willy. In insisting that his grandmother's cooking is not just flawed, it is so bad that it's not fit for humans, Willy, rather unheroically, becomes notable in the family for his insults.

The dog food story suggests a genre of joking deeply rooted within the African American tradition. Delores presents a grandson who has (somewhat precociously) already begun to master an important rhetorical skill. By valorizing such tales as the "Dog Food Dinner," Delores draws upon the culturally authorized capability to trade insults. Anthropologists and sociolinguists have long attended to this form of playful verbal virtuosity that has been cultivated in the African American community. Abrahams noted some decades ago: "Perhaps the clearest indication of the distinctiveness of the Black speech community lies in the use of speech in the pursuit of public *playing.* . . . Playing, in fact, is an important way in which one distinguishes oneself in public, and engaging in witty verbal exchanges is one important way of playing" (1974:241). Among children, this can be initiated as part of disputing (Goodwin 1990). Traditionally in the Black Oral Tradition, insults took the form of "the dozens"—riffs that were ritually aimed at someone's mother or other relatives (Labov 1972:304; Smitherman 1999). Speaking in the vernacular popular in the 1990s, Smitherman elaborates: "Literally speaking, when you 'dis' someone, you discount, discredit, disrespect that person—a dis is an insult. In the Black Oral Tradition, however, a dis also constitutes a verbal game, played with ritualized insults. The disses are purely ceremonial, which creates a safety zone. Like it's not personal, it's business—in this case, the business of playing on and with the Word" (1999:223).

In Delores's story, she attributes this verbal agility to Willy. He has evidently offered "dozens" insults not about someone else's mother (as would be proper) but about her, the most authoritative maternal figure in his household. In attributing this insult to Willy, Delores is encouraging him to cultivate a particular kind of skill that he will need in order to survive in the world of other children. The purpose of this kind of game, variously called "dissing," "signifyin," or "snaps," is one-upmanship. For this, it is a game "best played in a group of appreciative onlookers, who are secondary participants in the game" (Smitherman 1999:224).

As Sasha feared, when Willy grew older he became a regular target of teasing, not only by "harsh" children on the street or at school but within the family. Willy needs this capability for wit even to survive the taunts he gets by his cousins at home. His older cousins are quick to reprimand him by pointing out his "ugly face." Sasha's attempts to promote Willy's identity as a child special for his intelligence—not his facial scars—were severely challenged as he grew older. It was clear he was becoming more sensitive to his looks. By the time he was five, for example, when we asked him to draw a picture of himself (a common technique in our child interviews), he refused. "I can't draw me," he said. When asked why not, he replied, "I can't draw me cuz of my burns. I don't know how to draw my burns." He was happy to draw other members of his family, however.

Delores combats this self-consciousness in a manner very different than Sasha. Sasha's initial transformation of the home space—covering up all the mirrors—is reworked by Delores, who eases Willy into family routines where his quick wit can be highlighted. The point is not to hide his face (Sasha's instinct) but to learn how to show his face. Delores's Willy is the kind of boy who not only gets called "ugly" by his own family, he can use this insult to advantage to display his own superior wit. We can see this in the following exchange with his younger cousin Charles with whom he regularly squabbles. In this interchange, Willy provokes a fight to be captured "on camera" by Kim, one of the researchers on the project. The initial provocation occurs when, grinning, Willy suddenly tries to stick his fingers up Charles's nose. Charles squirms away as Kim looks on uncomfortably, wondering whether she should try to separate the boys. Willy does this in full awareness that he is being filmed and relies on Kim as audience.

Willy (to Kim): Watch this, he don't like people digging in his nose.

Kim: I wouldn't think so. I don't like people digging in my nose, do you?

Willy: Look, now look, he'll try to fight me. You see?

(Charles starts to swat Willy.)

Kim: Yup.
Willy: Stop Charles.
Charles: Shut up.
Willy: Whatchu say?
Charles: Shut up. That's what I—
Willy: (interrupts, more loudly) What did you say?
Charles: Just said, ugly.
Willy: Say (pauses with a glint in his eye) spell ugly.
Charles: (confused) Ugly? How do you spell?
Willy: No, there's a word called ugly. Spell it.

Charles confesses that he does not, in fact, know how to spell ugly, to Willy's delight. Although the two children are quite aware that the video camera is on them, these exchanges are common among the cousins. Willy's "ugliness" becomes a part of him that can be exploited in their rough-and-tumble play where everyone's vulnerabilities provide fodder in battles of one-upmanship. Though Willy is regularly taunted by Charles for his "ugliness," he proves to have his own resources for rebuttal and even instigation, showcasing Charles's ignorance of spelling. Willy's skill here is not only a matter of mastering a form of verbal play but also necessary in a child's world in which he must learn to stand up for himself in whatever disputes arise with other children. In Goodwin's exquisite ethnography of African American children's play and social organization, she noted that children themselves believed it important that they be able to fight their own battles without assistance. "Indeed, requiring the assistance of an adult is treated as a form of cowardice and can result in extensive ridicule. Children state that the intervention of adults in their disputes is unnecessary" (1990:156).

One could trace Willy's skill and his willingness to play such games to the training that Delores has provided through her insistence on family narrations of, for example, the Dog Food Dinner. Willy is neither hero nor victim but someone who can give as good as he gets. Here, the home emerges as a sanctuary, not in the way Sasha hopes for and sometimes euphemistically portrays it—a place in which her son is safe from being insulted—but one in which safety comes from being able to take up a "subject position" of the disfigured boy and play with it, even use it to advantage, in a game of jokey teasing.

TRANSCENDENCE, FRAGILITY, AND THE EVERYDAY

In this chapter and the previous one I have considered events in Delores's family as a way to offer a transcendent and experimental portrait of the moral ordinary. Everyday routines figure as both cultural resource and precarious achievement. Willy's accident initiates a process of moral learning for Sasha that could be described in the vocabulary of self-crafting—a self in need of tutoring.[3] However, the apprenticeship imaginary leaves out a crucial element of her moral task. She must learn things that are not predetermined in the kind of well-specified way that this imaginary tends to presume. The whole project of moral becoming illuminated here concerns how to live *this* particular life, to judge the best good within *these* singular circumstances. "Chance" opens new futures and forecloses others. Sasha need not have had to learn to cultivate the particular virtues she has in order to be a good mother; the accident has propelled her into acquiring new strengths and compassion. Some possibilities abruptly disappear. She might have been able to continue to develop her career as a dancer if her son had not been hurt.

As Willy grows older, he is no longer the same center of family concern. New family tragedies arise that once again threaten family love and reveal its limits. Most devastating for Willy was the incarceration of his mother Sasha, the death of Delores, and two months later, the murder of his beloved cousin Leroy, when Willy was just nine years old. Leroy was shot and killed in his front yard while Willy stood just next to him. The two boys had been very close, with Leroy often acting as his protector. What can small family routines offer in the face of these crushing blows? I offer one final scene at Leroy's funeral where Willy gives a speech. I return to that moment, still so vivid in my mind.

During Leroy's funeral service, when (as is customary) there is a time reserved for people from the floor to come up to speak, Willy stands and makes his way to the front of the church. He is the only one among his young cousins in the household who chooses to do so. The church is packed with at least two hundred people as he turns to face the congregation. Several other friends and older family members have already spoken, recounting their memories of Leroy, reading poems they have written, or offering carefully prepared speeches. Then Willy takes the microphone. His voice unwavering, he extemporaneously narrates a series of short stories about Leroy and the trouble the two of them got up to, everyday trouble that involved teasing sisters or trying to boss each other around. Willy recounts the ongoing trading of insults, mock battles, and trickery that were part of his relationship with Leroy, the way he would "dare" his cousin (more than twice his size) to come get him while racing to lock himself in the bathroom. He was the only speaker that day who made those of us in the audience laugh. Willy concluded his speech by saying to us, but also to Leroy, lying in the casket a few feet away: "*Well, that's my story about Leroy. My man, I love you.*" I was astonished at this young man, small for his age and still visibly scarred, a boy who had witnessed his cousin gunned down just a few days earlier, able to face a crowded church and know how to hold an audience with ease. In thinking about it later, I suddenly remembered the dog food story that Delores had told so many years before and the way that learning how to trade insults could become not only a means for defending yourself but an expression of family love.

CHAPTER 5

Moral Tragedy

The Perils of a Superstrong Black Mother

One of the most important endeavors of human practical reason will be to ask in a practical way (not a deep metaphysical way) about the relationship between natural necessity and human effort. . . . [Tragedies] typically invite us to sharpen our deliberative faculties in just this way, learning how to make the valuable distinction between . . . the sphere of chance and fate, and the sphere of justice.

—Nussbaum (2009:222)

Dotty's daughter Betsy has sickle cell anemia.[1] This genetic disease can be quite mild or, in cases like Betsy's, it can become so severe that it precipitates medical crises that are life threatening. It is not the kind of illness that one can necessarily detect from a person's physical appearance, but it can radically alter a person's life. In Betsy's case, it has meant repeated trips to the emergency room during acute episodes, weekly overnight stays in the hospital to receive blood transfusions, managing a host of medications, living with pain that is chronic and can become excruciating, having compromised lungs (a condition often associated with severe cases of the anemia), and living with the unpredictable and troublesome side effects of her many medications.

Dotty has had to learn how to manage this disease for her daughter. Although she sometimes receives help from her mother in caring for Betsy, and at times Dotty and Betsy have lived with her, she and her mother do not see eye to eye in how to raise her daughter, and Dotty prefers to have her own place. Part of learning to care for Betsy has involved mastering a wide range of medical knowledge about the disease and becoming adept at getting needed attention from clinicians. This has sometimes meant following their instructions but it has also meant being willing to question and challenge their advice in light of her own understanding of her daughter's illness. When, as a baby, her daughter was first diagnosed, Dotty hoped the clinicians could just "fix" her, she remembers with an ironic laugh. Several years later, she knows better. This is going to be a lifelong issue for Betsy, and it has changed Dotty's life in dramatic ways. She has had to postpone her own dreams of going back to school, and she has deferred her desire to explore romantic relationships or, as she has put it bluntly, to "have a life." She has had to become skilled at challenging clinicians when she believes them to be wrong, doing so in a way that doesn't make them so defensive they dismiss and ignore her. She learned this the hard way after she was "kicked out" of a community hospital close to her home where her daughter had been going for weekly transfusions. Although the hospital was convenient, it was small and staff did not know as much about sickle cell disease as the hospital where she took Betsy for her primary appointments, a well-staffed and preeminent teaching facility a two-hour drive from her house. Her attempts to navigate the two clinical sites and the necessity of being more directive about Betsy's care with the comparatively inexperienced staff at the community hospital created a series of escalating conflicts that she could not manage. Eventually the community hospital refused to admit her daughter. She learned some tough lessons about diplomacy from this experience. If she has become a "Loud Mom" during a confrontation, she has learned to return to the clinical staff she has challenged and thank them for their hard work on her daughter's behalf. She sometimes refers to herself as "Rambo Mom."

RAMBO MOM GOES INTO ACTION

I open onto a scene that has become part of ordinary life for them—another visit to the hospital to see a doctor about Betsy's latest health problems. Dotty, harried and tense, her beautiful face drawn with worry, leans against the wall of the examining room, waiting for the pulmonologist to arrive. Her daughter, nine years old at the time, is seated on the examining table, slumped, head down. She is reading a book. Soon Dr. Kesen comes in, hearty and cheerful. He is a large man, middle aged, with a smile that can warm a room, and he uses it to great effect. He briefly greets mother and child in a casual way. Though he is not Betsy's primary doctor (she mainly sees a hematologist), he knows them both. Betsy has had lung complications from birth, a common problem for those like her who have severe sickle cell anemia. Visits to the pulmon-ologist are not uncommon. Dr. Kesen turns jokingly to Betsy, who has continued to read her book, pulling her arms tight to her sides. Dotty laughs, though her laugh is tense, as he teases Betsy. I quote from a tran-script of this session, which was videotaped.

> *Dr. Kesen:* So, why've you got so sick? (He pauses.) That's what I'm sup-posed to find out, right?
>
> *Betsy:* [nods]
>
> *Dr. Kesen:* Yeah. You have high expectations, don't you? [Dotty laughs.] Okay, alright, so . . . (He pauses.) . . . because regrettably I don't remem-ber all the details of the things you sent me, why don't you give me a recap? [Dotty laughs.] (Now in a serious voice) I mean, I remember she was sick, but I don't remember . . .
>
> *Dotty:* (interrupting) Okay.
>
> *Dr. Kesen:* (teasing voice now, directed to Dotty) And I said that I was gonna solve it today.
>
> *Dotty:* (jokingly) You sure did, you're good.
>
> *Dr. Kesen:* No problem.
>
> *Dotty:* Uhhh, let's . . . here are the x-rays from the, the three illnesses, two illnesses? February's, July's . . . I only have the most recent x-rays for you.
>
> *Dr. Kesen:* (grinning) Ah, forget it then.
>
> *Dotty:* (laughs) But it's the same–
>
> *Dr. Kesen:* This is a comedy, right?
>
> *Dotty:* Yes. Absolutely.
>
> *Dr. Kesen:* Right. (He looks carefully through the x-rays she presents to him, going over them as they both stand and review them together.)
>
> *Dr. Kesen:* (referring to the x-rays) Have you seen these?
>
> *Dotty:* Oh yeah. Dr. Carter went over them with me Friday, and he said, not impressed. (She chuckles.)
>
> *Dr. Kesen:* He's not impressed?
>
> *Dotty:* Yeah, they are not acute chest he said.
>
> *Dr. Kesen:* Oh, okay, well that's good.
>
> *Dotty:* He believes they are asthma.
>
> *Dotty:* I'll bring it in to you, so you can look at them and . . .
>
> *Dr. Kesen:* (Dotty and Dr. Kesen look at the x-rays together, which Dr. Kesen has put up on the x-ray viewer) She was hospitalized for this?
>
> *Dotty:* Yes, yes. On all of these occasions, she was transfused, um, on all of these occasions she had this retro-sternal chest pain, leg pain and headache.

Dr. Kesen: Really?

Dotty: Uh huh. On the July pictures she was diagnosed. They said she had microplasma pneumonia.

Dr. Kesen: Really?

Dotty: Yeah, but Dr. Carter said—

Dr. Kesen: By the blood test?

Dotty: Yeah. He said, you can't go by that because once you get it, you know, you could have the antibodies.

Dr. Kesen: Right, that's true.

Dotty: They treated her with Biaxin and sent her out—sent the taxi.

The jocularity of the earlier exchange has disappeared as mother and doctor gaze together at the three x-rays she has brought. They are moving into treacherous terrain, and not just medically speaking. When Dr. Kesen asks her if she has "seen these," he also seems to imply that he wonders how she has been informed about them. This is not a small question, for it suggests the tricky border passage the two of them will have to negotiate. Dotty tells him yes, she has seen them because Dr. Carter, Betsy's hematologist and primary physician, went over them with her a few days earlier ("last Friday"). She adds, "And he said, he's 'not impressed.'" She has given the pulmonologist a critical piece of information. If she is here in this office to see the lung specialist, this is not on the recommendation of Betsy's primary physician. Quite the opposite—he is "not impressed" because he does not believe the x-rays point to "acute chest." His diagnosis is something much more benign. It is simply Betsy's asthma that is creating chest pain. This conclusion, although serious, is chronic. Nothing urgent is happening here.

It becomes obvious at this point that Dotty has come to Dr. Kesen because she does not completely trust Dr. Carter's diagnosis and wants a second opinion from the specialist. She has delicately, but in no uncertain terms, presented a political challenge to Dr. Kesen. He will not want to go against a fellow clinician, especially one who works in the same hospital and who he sees regularly. And yet, he knows Dotty knows this as well and will be watching to see if he takes her concern seriously or simply tries to placate her so as not to ruffle the feathers of a colleague.

He first approaches this by asking her a series of questions, relying upon her to give him a synopsis of medical events surrounding the mysterious chest pain. In the midst of this exchange, in which he has not only been challenged to solve the mystery, but also to navigate treacherous waters that have placed him between Dotty and Dr. Carter, Dr. Kesen suddenly changes the tone. He turns back to Betsy and introduces another comic routine. He begins with an innocuous setup.

> *Dr. Kesen:* (suddenly turning to Betsy) Have you seen your x-rays before?
>
> *Betsy:* (Looks up, startled, from her book. She shakes her head no.)
>
> *Dr. Kesen:* Well, you looking now?
>
> *Betsy:* (She nods yes.)

And with that, the joke proper begins. With mock seriousness, Dr. Kesen announces he will test her "in a minute" about the organs in her body that her x-rays show. He asks, "Does she want to try to guess some of them?" Yes, she nods gamely.

> *Dr. Kesen:* Okay . . . I'm gonna test you in a minute. Okay? You ready? What grade are you in?
>
> *Betsy:* Fourth.
>
> *Dr. Kesen:* Fourth? Have you learned about uh, like organs in the body?
>
> *Betsy:* No.
>
> *Dr. Kesen:* None? I bet you can guess, what some of them are. You wanna try?
>
> (Betsy nods.)
>
> *Dr. Kesen:* Okay. (He places the x-rays against the light.) But if you're wrong, it's okay, we won't punish you or anything. Okay? What's that big L? (Dr. Kesen points to the letter "L" on one of the x-rays of the screen while asking this.)
>
> *Betsy:* Left.
>
> *Dr. Kesen:* Left, that's right. That's not part of you. Which is, I guess, a good thing.

Dotty laughs and even Betsy smiles. He continues in this fashion, coaching her when she is unsure, until she correctly identifies her backbone, collar bone (she has trouble with this one), and arm bones. As he points to them on the x-ray, he also touches her body so that she can feel the correspondence. He gives her the kinesthetic evidence that what is on the screen is not alien (like the "Left") but actually part of her. It is as though he were giving her back her body.

> *Dr. Kesen:* Okay. So, what do you think this is?
>
> *Betsy:* Backbone?
>
> *Dr. Kesen:* Backbone, right. Okay, what do you think these are? I just pointed to 'em, your collarbones. Feel 'em right here? Now, got it? Okay, good, alright. Okay, what do you think these are?

Betsy: My arm bones.

Dr. Kesen: Your arms, very good, excellent. Now listen, if you answer two more right, you got my job, okay? You got a bunch of patients you gotta see this afternoon.

(Betsy laughs.)

Dr. Kesen: Okay, you ready? You're up for it? Okay, what do you think this is? (There is a pause while Dr. Kesen waits for her answer.) In the middle of your chest. (Another long pause.) It pumps blood around.

Betsy: (shrugging her shoulders) My heart?

Dr. Kesen: Absolutely! Excellent. Okay, what do you think these two black things are?

Betsy: My ribs?

Dr. Kesen: No, these are ribs. The bigger black things . . . inside.

Betsy: My lungs?

Dr. Kesen: Your lungs. Excellent, okay you got my job!

(Dotty and Betsy laugh.)

Dr. Kesen: Alright, we'll just go over the patients you have to see a little bit later, okay? Is that right? Okay. Alright. First of all, I'm sorry, you gotta have fun here occasionally. Okay.

He continues. Evidently this is not a mere (pretend) school test for a fourth grader, but a grown-up doctor's test. When he announces, "Alright, listen, you answer two more right, you got my job. Okay?" Dotty starts to relax, chuckling, and Betsy rewards him with a wide, shy smile. By the time he has concluded his "fun," everyone is laughing.

In this teasing exchange, Dr. Kesen has not only turned the tables—the patient becomes the doctor—but he has spoken to a deep-seated longing in Dotty. Dotty has had to undergo her own transformative journey as mother to this critically ill child. She has wanted to return to school for a nursing degree. Dotty would have preferred to become a doctor and would have considered this if her financial circumstances had been different and if she hadn't had a very sick daughter to care for. As a single mother of a very ill child, she does not hope for this, but she does hope she might be able to get a college-level nursing degree. And yet, because her daughter suffers from so many acute episodes, and she works full time to support the two of them, this is a dream continually postponed. She has signed up for night classes again and again, and even moved back in with her mother to help care for Betsy, in order to try to realize this dream. But Betsy has always gotten too sick and she has had to abandon her classes partway through the term.

This playful moment invokes an even deeper dream, speaking to a hope that Dotty hardly dares speak about. Until recently, children as sick as Betsy rarely lived past their early twenties. But thanks to recent medications, even those severely afflicted have been able to live until their early forties. "Maybe Betsy will become a doctor," Dotty has told us a few times over the years, in her more optimistic moments. This wish speaks not only to Betsy's intelligence and Dotty's insistence that she get to school as much as possible, but to her hope to have a daughter who is well enough and lives long enough to have such a chance. Dotty expresses her longing for a child whose long acquaintance with the medical world will permit her to have goals as arduous as this. And in one fantasy moment, Dr. Kesen not only enacts this hope, he even suggests that it is not mere foolishness. In fact, he also teaches Betsy something about how to "read" her body in an x-ray. And she does pass this test.

Although Dr. Kesen cannot quite know the dreams he has invoked, he can see that he has put this worried mother more at ease. Perhaps she has even come to trust him a little, and it is her trust he needs before he tells her his medical opinion of what is going on with Betsy. Turning his attention once again to Dotty, he is ready to give his diagnostic announcement, one that accords with Dr. Carter's. He then proceeds to give her clinical evidence to support his claim, pointing to the x-rays as he makes his case. In acute chest, he tells her, "the lungs are white, and these are not white." He goes on to underscore what Dr. Carter has told her, "which I actually agree with him on," he says, that the x-rays of Betsy's lungs show evidence of asthma.

> *Dr. Kesen:* Okay, so basically, what Dr. Carter was saying which I actually agree with him on, is the diaphragm's a little flattened here, you see?
>
> *Dotty:* Yeah.
>
> *Dr. Kesen:* Usually they're a little more like that. Which is called hyperinflation, which we see, if you have like asthma or obstruction in the airways because you have more trouble breathing out than breathing in, so your lungs get bigger. Make sense? So, I would agree, that really these . . . don't show acute chest. Now there might well be a little bit of pneumonia, kind of in this area, so the antibiotics were fine. . . . (He looks at a later x-ray, commenting.) Now this is the February one, and this one's better . . . so that's good.

Satisfied that he has solved the diagnostic puzzle, he returns to Betsy, who has gone back to reading her book. Dr. Kesen tells her that they will be "fiddling" with her asthma treatment.

In what follows, Dr. Kesen initiates a third joking sequence, this time directed to Dotty. "Now has Dr. Carter called me any bad names in front of you?" he asks. Dotty laughs in surprise. "No!" she replies emphatically, shaking her head. Dr. Kesen tells her that he is "chairman of the committee that has to approve all the new research studies, to make sure they don't harm people." Dotty also knows Dr. Carter is carrying out some experimental research protocols and he would have come up against Dr. Kesen's review committee. Dr. Kesen continues, his voice serious now as Dotty listens intently, "So, a lot of people in the hospital . . . they don't like regulatory type people." "No, they don't," Dotty agrees. With this, Dr. Kesen returns to his explanation of what he sees on the x-rays. Dotty mentions that she wants Betsy to participate in a clinical trial Dr. Carter will be conducting. "Good for you," he replies.

What is Dr. Kesen doing here? Having provided clinical evidence to support his agreement with a fellow clinician, he introduces another kind of evidence, namely, that doctors don't necessarily band together. All is neither homogeneous nor harmonious in the clinical world, he intimates with wry humor. He conspiratorially tells Dotty that she should "inform" on her daughter's primary physician. His suggestion, of course, violates all sorts of implicit moral codes—especially the one that says doctors are loyal to one another in front of their patients. By joking in this way, Dr. Kesen announces that he (a "regulatory type," no less) is willing to violate such a basic code.

His humor carries another message: that he is the sort of doctor who acts as a kind of guardian over patients, trying to protect them from harm that could be inflicted through his colleagues' research efforts. It might seem that with all these appeals to his trustworthiness, Dotty would accept Dr. Kesen's affirmation of Dr. Carter's diagnosis (asthma). But this is not the case.

He reiterates that he agrees with Betsy's pulmonologist that although the x-rays show signs of asthma, this is not something more serious. In response to his repeated declaration, "So I would agree that these are not acute chest," Dotty simply objects. She does not know what is going on, is willing to trust that the doctors are right about this diagnostic possibility, but she is certain that *something* is wrong. She persists doggedly, politely but with arms pressed tightly to her sides. "But clinically, I mean her symptoms, she's very, very sick you know." Dr. Kesen demurs. "Well, asthma can make you sick." But Dotty continues, trying to impress upon him the gravity of the sickness, providing her own clinical evidence. Betsy has "been in there [the hospital], on morphine," she points out. "Well, okay," Dr. Kesen replies, "but the morphine is—I don't think it's for her lungs. It's probably for [he pauses, considering]—you said she was having leg pains?" "Yeah, well, we're still trying to figure out what that is," Dotty tells him. "Like in the hospital, they had her on, Fentanyl." (Fentanyl is a much more powerful opiate than morphine.) This stops Dr. Kesen short. "Jeez," he says in surprise. From here, the discussion shifts into what might be causing this level of pain, which Dr. Kesen does not believe could be Betsy's lungs. Could it be the leg pain Betsy has been experiencing? Dotty notes, "We're still trying to figure out what that is," and mentions Dr. Carter's hypothesis, that it is something "neuromuscular." "She [Betsy] has it now," Dotty adds. Dr. Kesen turns to Betsy to find out about the pain, asking her questions about how and where she feels it.

The rest of the session (about ten more minutes) continues this puzzling process as the pulmonologist proceeds to ask Betsy a series of questions about the nature of her pain (sharp, dull, or tingling) and where exactly in her body she is feeling it. Dotty offers more information, a kind of walking chart review, as she summarizes more of Betsy's recent pain problems, her trips to the emergency room, and the treatment she was given in the emergency room. Dotty tells of these emergency trips to the hospital not simply as dramatic events but, more difficult still, as part of a long, terrible process that brings no ultimate relief. Notice the change in tense with which she describes one such incident. It moves from specific past to timeless present. The drama of an acute episode is not extraordinary at all, her tense shift implies, but an ever-present horror embedded in everyday life: "But that night, around three o' clock in the morning, she woke up telling me her chest hurt and I just took her straight in to the ER. And by that time, she just went down. . . . her stats dropped too around that time. They always get lower one or two points and you know, by the time I get in the ER, two hours later, she's on oxygen, you know?" She sighs.

THE SUPERSTRONG BLACK MOTHER AS MORAL TRAGEDY

This clinical exchange reveals how enormously well versed Dotty is about her daughter's medical situation and her ability to draw the doctor into an in-depth discussion of medical issues. Clinicians at this hospital are not as respectful of all parents as they are of Dotty. She has earned special privileges with them. She has learned over the years not only to become extremely medically knowledgeable but to also become highly vigilant. Like a critical care clinician, she watches the subtlest signs to monitor impending crises. As one of the physicians put it, discussions with Dotty are "almost like talking to another doctor." And yet, Dotty feels herself morally endangered by exchanges such as the one with Dr. Kesen. Why is this so? She may have become a strong and skilled mother, but this is not enough. Through her practice of care for Betsy, Dotty has come to embody the subject position and virtues associated with a Superstrong Black Mother. Paradoxically, it is her very success at cultivating the virtues necessary for caring for her daughter within the particular circumstances of her daughter's illness that create moral problems for her. To illustrate the depth of the moral peril she finds herself in, I turn to the ancient consideration of moral tragedy.

The human vulnerability to fate was especially epitomized in Greek tragedy. The dramas of Greek antiquity had an enormous influence on its moral philosophy and caused considerable philosophical debate. "Greek tragedy shows good people being ruined because of things that just happen to them, things that they do not control," Nussbaum remarks (1986:25). This in itself is not news—everyone recognizes this unhappy fact of life. However, Greek dramas paid special attention to what might be called *moral tragedy,* situations in which good people came to act in ways they would otherwise reject, to do bad things, because of circumstances they did not initiate and whose consequences they did not or could not foresee. More controversial, however, the moral tragedies showed good people acting in ways that they consciously knew were bad because they were caught in a tragic conflict between two incommensurable ethical claims. "Tragedy tends, on the whole, to take such situations very seriously," Nussbaum goes on to explain. "It treats them as real cases of wrong-doing that are of relevance for an assessment of the agent's ethical life. Tragedy also seems to think it valuable to dwell upon these situations, exploring them in many ways, asking repeatedly what personal goodness, in such alarming complications, is" (1986:25). MacIntyre points out that it was particularly the ancient Greek playwright Sophocles who argued through his tragedies that life can present us with insolvable moral dilemmas, with "rival and incompatible claims upon us. . . . Our situation is tragic in that we have to recognize the authority of both claims" (1981:134).

Already the radical implications of this pre-Socratic worldview represented in Greek tragedies created problems for the philosophy of antiquity. Even in antiquity there were philosophical "opponents of luck" who argued "that which we ourselves control is in every case sufficient to secure" it (Nussbaum 1986:322).[2] Some philosophers eschewed the moral implications of such tragedies in the name of reason, arguing that "stories depicting the collisions of competing claims of right are repugnant to reason, since they assert a contradiction" (Nussbaum 1986:25). These ancient philosophical opponents of luck also argued that goods (including other people) were commensurable, Nussbaum contends. This allowed the possibility for weighing various goods by some universal standard or measure—offering an essentially quantitative solution to conflicts among goods. This path toward adjudication among competing goods would be systematically and quantitatively developed in European moral philosophy in the eighteenth and nineteenth centuries. This rejection of moral incommensurability and the triumph of reason over circumstance is, of course, a hallmark of the moral philosophy of modernity.

However, many contemporary neo-Aristotelian moral philosophers have embraced not only the idea that reason cannot necessarily lead one out of such quandaries, but that the kind of moral predicament that may lead a good person to do bad things for reasons out of that person's control is, in fact, part of the human condition. Thus tragedy, from an Aristotelian perspective, is quite specifically bound up with moral dilemmas. It is not to be equated merely with an unhappy ending for it is an unhappy ending of a very particular sort. In this neo-Aristotelian view, since moral considerations cannot be determined from any universal standpoint alone but must be judged in terms of the particularities of each situation, actors are often faced with difficult moral choices. It might be presumed that to minimize such peril, any hoped for "best good" ought to be reduced to a good that one could reasonably expect to attain. But Aristotle disagreed. He believed that human flourishing requires the pursuit of goods that fall well outside of human control, especially the control of a single moral agent. A best good might require taking a course of action during which we are not only highly unsure of our success, but that could engender a morally tragic outcome.

To highlight how a revived Aristotelian version of virtue ethics and its portrait of the human condition can tell us something about Dotty's situation, I draw especially upon Nussbaum's analysis in her classic work, *The Fragility of Goodness* (1986). Here, she contrasts an Aristotelian picture from a "self-sufficing" and autonomous portrait of moral decision, deliberation, and action that was already a point of contention in ancient Greece. (She credits Plato with the self-sufficing version.) My purpose is not to rehash a 2,500-year-old debate, but to follow Nussbaum in emphasizing the importance of Aristotle's more vulnerable version of the moral.

DOTTY'S MORAL TRAGEDY

Where is the tragedy for Dotty? Paradoxically, Dotty's very clinical knowledge and adeptness is an indication of a tragic incommensurability at the heart of her effort to create a "good life" for herself and her daughter. Hers is a hard-won expertise. It has cost her and her daughter a great deal. It is not simply that the price of such clinical competence has been "no life" of her own or, for long stretches, a return to living with her own mother, with whom she has a rocky relationship. Most tragically, from Dotty's perspective, honing this medical gaze has separated her from her own child. The doctor may be able to draw Betsy in as a child, but this is a skill Dotty fears she has nearly lost. *This* is the price of her competence. She has become acutely attuned to Betsy's body, and especially to the treacheries of her body—the face of serious disease. But because of this, Dotty has become more and more blinded to her daughter's plight as just another little girl.

Dotty's immense medical expertise, her capabilities as a "border crosser" who travels knowledgably in the clinical world, and her cultivation of a vigilant clinical gaze that she has trained upon her daughter represent a cost that runs through her whole life and her child's life as well. Although Betsy's physicians see her situation as relatively "stable," for Dotty there is nothing "stable" about Betsy's life. Dotty is watching her child grow up with a combination of a serious lung disease and quite severe sickle cell. Her daughter has spent four days out of the week in the hospital since she was young and has had to be rushed to the emergency room periodically for acute pain episodes.

As Dotty has remarked despairingly, "What kind of life is this for a child?" Dotty and Betsy have little time together as mother and daughter without all of their interactions being constrained by hospital settings and by Betsy's enforced idleness as she lies in bed for hours during transfusions. Betsy has even less time to make friends and "to just be a child." Dotty rushes from work to the hospital and home again. She wants for her and Betsy to "experience life." Instead, she has a child who actually enjoys going to the hospital. "I mean she doesn't, she looks forward to going to the hospital. I think that's weird," Dotty says. When it comes to Wednesday night, Betsy will announce, "Tomorrow's Thursday. I get to go [to] the hospital, I get to sleep there, and I'm just looking forward. I'm so excited I'm going." Dotty shakes her head at the "weirdness" of a child who would come to find the hospital a place to look forward to.

Most painfully, she herself sometimes "forgets" that her daughter is her child and not her patient. She loses sight of how to "just be a mother." Dotty tells the following poignant story of one such moment of horrifying clarity, an experience of this kind of forgetting, of not seeing, blinded by her own medical gaze:

> Betsy went on the bus to camp. She started crying, right? She's sitting there, sobbing her little eyes out. And I'm like, "Betsy, what's wrong with you? What's the matter?" I'm looking at her, trying to figure out, "Why is she crying?" I don't understand it. She's going to have a great time. She's getting away from me. Why is she crying? And then it clicked with me. Oh, she's crying because she doesn't—she's gonna *miss* you. You know, it's one thing when you go together, it's one thing when I go. But it's another thing when she gets on the bus, and she goes, and she's gonna *miss* me. So that's why she's crying. I had to figure all this out in my brain, because I was just so separated from it all. And I looked, and I said, "Oh that's what it is" (laughs). So I had to connect with that, and then I sat down in a seat, and I said [to myself], "You know what? I need to put my arms around this girl and hold her. Let her know that I'll see her when she gets back. That's the appropriate response." Now most mothers would know that, right? Me? Because I'm just trying to figure out, well why is she crying? What's going on? Is she in pain? Is this happening? Is that happening? I'm trying to process all those things first. So there's a lag, or a delay. So when I finally realized it, I sat down in a chair, and then I held her. And I said, "Oh Betsy, I'll see you when you get back. You're gonna have a great time, you got all your friends. And you know it's okay to miss me, but it's alright, you know. I'll be right here, and I'll see you when you get back." Had to keep telling her that. And I said, "Okay, I'm gonna go now. See you later." And I get off the bus, and you know, and I go. And she was fine. But it really, it really hit home for me. I'm like, my God, you know, I really, really am detached.

Dotty has also had to develop other skills that equip her to fight for her child's care. She has learned how to be a "Rambo," a skill she did not possess initially. But this can also detach her from her daughter. She worries that she is becoming the sort of person who, like Rambo, is more adept at fighting than at holding her daughter, an issue that she has talked over with the psychologist she now sees. On the one hand, this is a skill she needed to cultivate. She needed to learn to confront, to fight for care, or to simply challenge clinicians when their perceptions did not accord with hers, as she does in a very clear way with Dr. Kesen. She may not sound like Rambo with her persistent but well-measured questioning, but this is how it feels to her. On the other hand, she is worried about the kind of person she is becoming as a result, a mother who spends so much time and emotional energy as "Rambo" that she loses her kinder, softer qualities and anger takes over her whole life. We can see her fear of this in her description of a recent conflict with a nurse who she believed was dismissing Betsy's pain:

> I just blew up. And I really didn't care what people thought at the time. I didn't care what I was doing, how I was act- I just didn't care. I was so angry. And I remember being, just full of it. Just so angry that if the woman [the nurse] had been standing in front of me, I would've snapped her neck. That's how mad I was.

Dotty can see that this "Rambo Mom" is difficult for Betsy as well:

> Right now, she [Betsy] doesn't want to have Mommy yelling at everyone on the planet. She wants her mommy. And I have to be able to switch from being, you know, "let's get this handled" to this other thing, that, you know, "she needs me now" type deal. And it's very hard to switch between the two. And that's part of that problem, like how do you turn it off? How do you turn off, you detach from it and say, you know, "I'm gonna detach from this whole situation and try to get this done, get this resolved so she can get good care." And how do I [also] be that mommy that has to, you know, sit there and put your arms around the child, and hold them?

The sheer relentlessness of Betsy's condition is sometimes almost unbearable for Dotty:

> Betsy has a chronic illness. And part of the problem with that is, someone says to you, chronic illness—you have such a hard time dealing with it as a parent, because it's not like having cancer, where three years from now, everything's over with. But when you have chronic illness, you have to come to terms with the fact that your child will continually, continually continue to be getting sick. And you never do. And I never have.

Dotty sees herself as cultivating virtues, like her Rambo-ness, that may be essential for times when she has to wage war but are completely at odds with those virtues that allow her to easily recognize a daughter sobbing on the camp bus who just needs a mommy to hold her. These are very difficult virtues to reconcile; perhaps they are even incommensurable, Dotty fears. From this moral vantage point, we can look at Dotty's situation as forcing her to live out an ongoing moral tragedy. For her, there is no one "best good" kind of mother to be, however strong she is able to become. There is no utilitarian calculus that will solve her problem. Nor is there some universal or Archimedean perspective from which to judge the ultimate best good. Her particular mothering task, caring for a medically fragile child, has compelled her on numerous occasions to "go into battle" with clinicians when she has judged her daughter at risk. Rambo may be an excellent warrior, but what kind of mother would he make? How can he tell when a child just needs to be held because she is going off to camp for the first time?

Dotty's decision to pursue a highly risky experimental procedure exemplifies with particular force the kind of moral agony she was experiencing. Her pained recognition that medical stability (to the extent Betsy even has it) comes at such a terrible cost propels Dotty to consider this dangerous option.

MORAL EXPERIMENTS WITH A RISKY CLINICAL SURGERY

For several years, Dotty has been trying to find out whether Betsy might be a candidate for a bone marrow transplant. When Betsy was nine, just at the time of the clinic visit I described earlier, Dotty began to seriously inquire about this possibility with Dr. Carter, the hematologist who has been treating Betsy since she was three years old. Dotty has had numerous discussions with him about this operation. If successful, a bone marrow transplant would rid Betsy of sickle cell disease. However, in even considering this option, Dotty finds herself caught in yet another moral dilemma, having to choose between two conflicting "best goods." One best good—a conservative attempt to keep Betsy medically stable—is undermined by another best good, taking a more high-risk medical intervention that could allow Betsy (and Dotty) to lead very different lives. This high-risk operation (if successful) might also alleviate a life that is not stable at all, but is punctuated by pain crises that can occur at any time and spiral into life-threatening emergencies in a matter of minutes.

An Aristotelian framework offers an important basis for understanding Dotty's struggles over the best good as she considers the option of a bone marrow transplant. Her decision to pursue this risky procedure— against the medical advice of the clinicians who treat Betsy—underscores the potential frailties of action: its riskiness, its necessarily social and interdependent nature, and its tragic possibilities. To further illustrate, I contrast her position with the moral reasoning that guides the clinicians who treat Betsy, especially Betsy's primary one, Dr. Carter, the hematologist. Contrasting their perspectives illuminates the way that Dotty is responding to a situation she finds morally incommensurable and why this view is not shared by the clinical staff.

Dotty's insistence on considering the transplant option is part of a long quest for a cure for Betsy. She realizes that she is hoping big, but this is as she puts it, her "mission statement." She has not only been risky in her dreaming, but also in her attitude toward high-risk clinical procedures. It is here, especially, that she and Dr. Carter have often parted company. Nowhere has this been as evident as in their intense discussions over the possibility of a transplant operation. Dr. Carter has told Dotty that he will not do such a transplant and if she decided that she wanted to find another hospital to do it, he "would tell her, that I wouldn't support it." When we interviewed him about his position he explained, "The data is that it's more dangerous. This is what Dotty is struggling with. It's very difficult, you know. She wants her kid not to have sickle cell disease. So do I, but at what risk?" He supports his view by noting that for some time Betsy has been doing well medically, given the severity of her sickle cell disease and other complications. "Overall, she's, from a medical standpoint, she's pretty much been . . . stable the whole time. And so she keeps getting these lung episodes which I'm not really sure are acute chest but you know, I think she's been stable and she's been growing."

We asked him if Betsy has been getting better. "No," he concedes, but repeats that she has been stable. Stability might sound as though nothing is happening, but in fact stability is itself a complex clinical achievement. Betsy is a medically fragile child, one who has had a series of life-threatening acute episodes in the early years of her life until Dotty heard about Dr. Carter and took Betsy to his sickle cell clinic for treatment. She became stable only under his care. He contrasts Betsy's medical condition with those he might be willing to perform a transplant on—children so sick that one might as well try. "You sort of do them on patients that are, you think you're gonna lose if you don't and she's [Betsy's] not in that condition at all." He offers an example to illustrate—and perhaps to justify—his own deliberation over this, where he is trying to get a patient to have a transplant:

> And I've got a teenage girl who's gonna die if we don't get rid of her sickle cell disease, she's probably gonna die in the next ten years. So I'm gonna try and sell to her, why don't you take a chance, you know? But you know, the problem with Betsy, according to her lung doc, she's gonna get better, her

lungs are gonna get better and she's getting better. And so, you know, that's not the kind of thing where I'm gonna say okay why don't you take a 10 percent chance of dying.

But Dotty is not satisfied with this. She wants more, hopes for more, both for her daughter and herself. She hopes for a cure from sickle cell and sees the experiments in bone marrow transplants as one possible route. She has talked to other doctors to get their opinions on the matter. Dotty decided to take a long trip to another major medical center in the San Francisco area to meet with a doctor (Dr. Lerner) whose medical team had been making great strides in sickle cell transplants. They had received a large NIH (National Institutes of Health) grant and were carrying out clinical trials in new procedures. She wanted to find out whether Betsy could be a candidate for this clinical trial, despite what Dr. Carter has told her.

She describes her meeting with the head of this transplant team and her excitement as a result of his encouragement: "I went down there to this medical center and spoke with him. And he looked at her [Betsy's] history and he says, "Yeah she'd be a great candidate. Of course I felt this was almost, we're almost at the end of the road. We're almost there." But when she discusses this with Dr. Carter, he suggests that she has, in fact, misunderstood what the Oakland team told her. Dotty is crushed by Dr. Carter's response. She has paid a high price in her search for a "good" that seems to be within reach, only to be snatched away. Her response might be to close down her hopes, to constrict her desires so that she is less vulnerable. But this is not what she does. Instead, she continues to propose the possibility of a transplant, looking into experimental unrelated donor transplants that are taking place in other highly regarded medical centers. She continues to bring this and other possibilities to Dr. Carter.

When it comes to the issue of taking risks versus constricting desires to what one can control, it is clear that Dr. Carter opts for the latter as far as possible. He resists the tragedy of Betsy's situation, as revealed in his language. He can keep her "safe" for ten years, and he does not veer into the murky and troublesome question of whether this is a kind of safety that gives Betsy or her mother a life worth living. In his role as physician, he works to constrict his own desires and those of Dotty and Betsy as well so that "ten more years" of safety may serve as a kind of happy ending.

It is easy to see that the "end" Dotty pursues cannot be hers alone but requires immense cooperation and coordination with others. There are, of course, political and economic issues of who will pay for such an operation. But there is the prior question of whether she can convince others—especially Dr. Carter—to investigate the possibility of this transplant. Dotty tries to make clear to Dr. Carter that she values his opinion and they are "in this together" in treating Betsy. When Dr. Carter told her he was not in fact comfortable and was unwilling to condone this surgery, Dotty grew very uneasy. She was not prepared to take a chance on her own judgment and disregard his. If this could not be a communally defined best good, she was not sure she could pursue it. She explains why Dr. Carter's approval is so important to her. It is not simply because of his expertise but also because of something much more, his friendship, his kinship even, to use Dotty's language: "And I don't want to move unless I know that he would be, it's kind of like having a father, you know? You don't want to move unless you have his blessing type deal. And if I know he's okay I'll be fine because I also know that he's very conservative."

Although Dr. Carter is perceived by Dotty (and by us on the research team, I might add) as an extremely caring and concerned clinician, he does not enter into the same world of incommensurability that Dotty does. He continues to define the best good in essentially clinical terms, weighing the cost of pursuing one clinical strategy against another in light of an overarching idea of keeping Betsy as medically stable as possible. He does not face Dotty's problem, which is that the cost of this stability may be the cultivation of selves (Betsy's, her own, and her family's) that she finds deeply problematic, even morally compromised. It is significant here that the potential for an *ethical* tragic incommensurability does not figure into the clinicians' (especially Dr. Carter's) practical reasoning in the way it does for Dotty.

There are certainly ways that his view of the good is tailored to Betsy—she emerges as a *particular* "child." Although he thinks in terms of general probabilities, he also tries to put together the many medical issues that are special to Betsy. It is telling that he and Dr. Lerner stand for two hours in a hotel hall at a hematology conference, "weighing the odds" of a bone marrow transplant for her. However, he departs from the more radical implications of the practical reasoning that Dotty embraces. He shies away from the possibility that they might be facing an ethically tragic situation. His preferred good is unwaveringly to keep Betsy medically stable for the next ten years. He draws upon the language of probabilities and calculations in his deliberations, supporting his strong view that the important thing for this medically fragile child is to minimize risks and to rely upon conventional therapy. His faith in future scientific and technical discoveries supports his position as well. In deliberating about what is best for Betsy, Dr. Carter also banks on improvements in medical technology. He states, "There's a lot of hope for these kids" because "the whole transplant technology is improving all the time." He reasons that if he can keep Betsy stable, "a lot can happen in ten years, in terms of transplant [technology]" that could be helpful for Betsy, including the "ability to do an extended matching."

Unlike Dotty, who does face a situation of incommensurable goods, Dr. Carter relies heavily upon a canonical clinical discourse that largely precludes this kind of reflection. And although he recognizes that his experience is inevitably different from Dotty's, he is not prepared to see this decision as representing a choice between incommensurable moral ends. Rather, he assumes that she differs in her willingness to take this risk for her daughter because, despite her intelligence, she does not have the professional experience or expertise of the practiced clinician. We can hear this in the way he describes how Dotty assesses the situation versus transplant specialists like Dr. Lerner and himself, who have "twenty-five years treating this disease": "And if a guy whose career is transplant [Dr. Lerner] and another guy who's been doing twenty-five years treating this disease [speaking of himself] are haggling over what do we think is the right thing to recommend, to expect a mom who's very intelligent, no less intelligent than I am, but to come to grips with all of this, the fine points of these differences, you know?"

MORAL DELIBERATION AS EXPERIMENT

In the first chapter, the moral experiment I introduce occurs in physical space and time. The soccer game literally changes the rules of the game—it is visibly marked in the material and social space of the field. I have suggested in the introduction to chapter 3 that sometimes such experiments are less visible. To be recognized they must be placed within a larger temporal arc, and for this I introduced the narrative trope of the journey. Dotty introduces a morally laden thought experiment about signing her daughter up in a risky clinical trial surgery (a literal science experiment) that she eventually rejects. Although she might have pursued the surgery option, she finally lets it drop. However, there are many experimental moments along the way. She sets a new dialogue in motion among physicians, including the transplant surgeon in Oakland. She experiments with ways to induce the optimal conditions for conducting this thought experiment that includes three specialists. To facilitate this, she even makes a "road trip" to Oakland with Betsy and her mother. Dotty experiments not because of some optimistic "against all odds" vision of the future, but because what she sees ahead of her is so treacherous. The future she can envision, as far as the eye can see, promises a bleaker—morally bleaker—fate that will befall her and her daughter. It is these odds that she challenges, willing even to place the life of her daughter into a medically hazardous situation. In giving up this experiment and this hope, she sees herself and her daughter condemned to cultivate virtues that harm them morally. If her daughter must continue to live with this kind of physical precariousness, Dotty finds herself committed to a path of moral becoming that is as unwanted as it is necessary.

MORAL LESSONS

Certainly, Aristotle's views of the moral life cannot simply be adopted without significant amendment. Aristotle, a member of an elite, after all, gives us no sufficient account of the workings of power. He would not acknowledge Dotty as a moral subject. (She is not an Athenian, she is not male, etc.) Nor would her practice of motherhood correspond to the practices that he was concerned with—the creation of a polis by free Athenian men. His ethics lacks a "sociology" and a "history," as MacIntyre has complained. Anthropology has something crucial to offer here. Even philosophers advocating a "thick" version of the moral self tend to offer highly truncated hypothetical examples or exemplars drawn from literature to work out their general claims. Anthropologists are able to engage such claims with something else—a kind of ethnographic "messiness" that provides resistance to abstractions and a continued insistence on attending to local cultural discourses.

What can Dotty's situation teach us? I suggest three lessons that complicate the picture we get from neo-Aristotelian philosophy. First, her situation suggests that moral tragedy is not simply an extreme possibility faced by persons in highly unusual circumstances (as in most Greek tragedies) but that it can have a more everyday face. Certainly her child's medical fragility is not exactly ordinary. But suffering, even suffering as acute as the sort Dotty faces, is all too prevalent throughout the world, as numerous anthropological accounts attest. Second, Dotty's dilemma suggests that the tragic dimensions of any particular situation may not be evident to all the participants in it. That is, it demonstrates that in the kinds of social worlds anthropologists study, the morally tragic may not be visible as a shared intersubjective interpretive framework: Dotty sees a tragedy where her daughter's doctors do not.

Finally, the anthropological insistence on the place of social discourses in shaping moral life locates questions of the human condition within particular cultural and historical spaces. It allows us to see that Dotty's dilemma is not simply shaped by some existential human condition or fate—a case of extremely "bad luck" in Greek terms. She is also shaped by a social history that has valorized a specific form of moral strength and tenacity in the face of adversity and provided powerful ideals for what a good mother should look like. In considering her situation, we might ask if her tragedy is absolutely necessary. Couldn't something be humanly done to alter the situation that parents and children like Dotty and Betsy face? Is this all a matter of fate and chance, or does justice play some part in it?

The social locatedness of her tragedy might seem far removed from the tragedies we have inherited from antiquity in which protagonists appear to be simply doomed to their fates. However, Nussbaum offers a different view in a fascinating essay in which she challenges Bernard Williams's picture of moral tragedy. Williams, whose work I have already drawn upon, took Greek tragedies very seriously, helping to reintroduce them to contemporary moral philosophy. Nussbaum notes appreciatively that he "makes an admirably lucid argument against various condescending progressivist interpretations of Greek culture, putting to rest, once and for all, the tired allegation that the early Greeks had no concept of deliberation and choice and a primitive notion of agency" (Nussbaum 2009:214). However, she adds, he fails to recognize a crucial function of these plays, namely to prompt moral deliberation around specific timely issues for the audiences who came to see them performed.

She suggests that "one of the valuable contributions of Greek tragedy to ethical thought is in fact a subtle process of deliberation about luck and bad human behavior, as we are again and again led to ask ourselves, 'What, in the terrible events we witness, is sheer luck and necessity, and could not have been otherwise? What, by contrast, is human folly, rapacity, and negligence, and could possibly have been otherwise?'" (2009:215). In order to understand their deliberative qualities, they must be understood not as texts denuded from the historical situation of the audience but rather as living performances that were directed to audiences who were also caught by these questions in contemplating their society and its actions. If tragedies provide us material to view the darkest side of life, what Williams calls the "horrors," this need not point toward an existential resignation. It can prompt scrutiny of what might have prevented such horrors. Nussbaum makes it clear that this was part of their purpose. The plays were performed at civic festivals. They were a central part of a civic religion that gave Athenian citizens an opportunity to engage in collective communal deliberation about ethics. She describes this scene of performance:

> The way plays were produced (by companies of citizen actors, trained by yet other citizens), the way the spectators were seated (with pride of place given to young men on the verge of military service), the way plays were routinely assessed (with a strong emphasis on their ethical content), all this heightened the sense that the witnessing of a play was an occasion for solemn civic deliberation. The very structure of the theatre—an amphitheatre across which one could see the faces of one's fellow citizens, as one sat in the bright sunlight—promoted community awareness and discouraged a retreat into private thoughts about human catastrophe. It is now commonplace to underline the deliberative context of the tragedies, and to see them as part of Athens' elaborate construction of civic reason and civic friendship. (2009:222)

In Nussbaum's description it becomes clear how these tragedies are not only expressions of personal moral horrors or existential and implacable fate but of the very human forms of society that might have been otherwise. Greek society itself, with its warring behavior and its callous and needless cruelties, is often displayed as a villain in these tragedies. She offers a number of compelling examples of plays whose content was ostensibly about historical events but whose message was directed to political situations that were contemporary and analogous. In watching the tragic unfolding of past events, the Greek audience could be provoked to deliberate about their current political situations, ones where they could still make choices as a citizenry and change the course of unfolding events. Nussbaum is especially respectful of those plays that asked such questions as "What can . . . good people do in a world run by powerful bad people?" Well, they can love one another, she suggests. But "most of all, they can talk: they can name the wrongs done to them, accuse those who wrong them, and carry those accusations into the record of history" (2009:231).

I have concluded this chapter with a sustained meditation on Nussbaum's arguments because they have such relevance for Dotty's situation. She is not only an actor in a moral tragedy. She is also an observer of that tragedy. As a spectator, she can ask some of the questions that

Nussbaum tells us Greek tragedians asked. What can even relatively powerless good people do in the face of powers that are unjust or evil? Dotty may not be able to save the tragic situation with her daughter during these years, but as witness to how she has been morally caught, she can ask what it is about our society that her situation reveals and what could be done to change it. What does her dilemma reveal about societal racism and the lack of funding and research support for a "black" disease like sickle cell anemia? What does it teach about the lack of financial support for parents like her, who have to take on such an enormous part of the care of her child? About the flaws in the health care system? About the racially inflected stigmatization of children like her daughter who receive heavy doses of opiates in pain crises and are looked upon by some clinical staff as drug addicts, or "med seeking," as they say in the clinical world?

"I never thought I was black until my daughter was diagnosed with sickle cell," she once said. Hearing her, I recalled the words of Zora Neale Hurston, the famous African American anthropologist of decades ago who wrote, "I remember the very day I became colored." What Dotty was telling me was that she had never felt the press of her racial identity so oppressively and systematically as when caring for a child marked by this disease. She comes to be an observer not only of her personal plight but also of others afflicted by sickle cell disease. Perhaps she cannot avoid the family moral tragedy that she lives, but she might be able to do something to prevent or lessen the kinds of misfortunes that have befallen her and her child. This activist response is exactly the route she has taken.

CHAPTER 6

The Flight of the Blue Balloons

Narrative Suspense and the Play of Possible Selves

Things are kind of hazy
And my head's all cloudy inside
And I've heard talk of angels
I never thought I'd have one to call mine
—Unknown Song

Hold fast to dreams
For if dreams die
Life is a broken-winged bird
That cannot fly.
—Langston Hughes, *Dreams* (1994:32)

Many complaints have been leveled against the idea of a first person narrative self. I mentioned some of them in chapters 1 and 2. Challenges come from several quarters. They are not only a product of postmodern/ poststructuralist "death of the author" declarations but are also expressed by phenomenologists concerned that linking narrative so closely with a conception of the self is deeply misleading. These critiques made by scholars embracing a first person phenomenology are important to attend to in light of my own project. Two are recurrently voiced. One, a narrative self suggests too much coherence and a simple linear view of unfolding life. I noted in chapter 2 that the image so often associated with the narrative self—life as a journey—seems to reinforce this. The journey metaphor immediately evokes a linear path and a space–time relationship of before and after, earlier and later, nearer and farther. A second objection is that a narrative portrait of the self relies too heavily on a linguistic understanding of experience. It is too semiotic and does not do justice to the importance of embodied practices in one's self experience.

It is true that the image of a life as an unfolding story can easily over-simplify what it is like to experience life over time. An overly coherent self does seem to be to be implied by some virtue ethics philosophers. I have recommended that the remedy is to take narrative *more* rather than less seriously and look carefully at what this narrative-like quality of the self entails. Certainly, the experience of moral transformation has far greater complexity than a linear, coherent and tellable life story inti-mates. In other works, I have proposed that what makes narrative so compellingly linked to lived experiences is not its linear qualities so much as its suspenseful ones.[1] A better way to think about the narrative self is to attend to the play of parallel selves and parallel lives that are intrinsic to lived experience. This can be illuminated by a narrative portrait of the self that does justice to such temporal complexity. Lived time has its lines and measures, it marches forward, but these lines are often hazy, roads marked by signposts seen through a fog. Haziness may even be culti-vated, not in order to avoid seeing what is ahead, but in order to face it.

The people I describe in this book do not merely live out one life story; they find themselves in the unsure position of being situated among several possible plots and all at once. Strikingly, they may even *cultivate* such uncertainty, creating experiences and events that speak to multiple futures and multiple possible selves. This cultivation of an *experimental narrative self* is the topic of this chapter.[2] I paint a highly experiential and embodied picture of narrative re-envisioning here, examining how one mother, Andrena, tries to create a good life in the midst of peril and avert the threat of moral tragedy through the simul-taneous nurturing of multiple and mutually exclusive life plots.

THE PLAY OF POSSIBLE LIVES

Of everyone I have come to know in this study, I have been closest to Andrena. She died in 2004, just before Thanksgiving. Although I speak of her in a present tense, she is present only in that special sense of someone still alive for me. There was, I think, a natural affinity between us—a simi-larity of age and perhaps of temperament. But the friendship that grew between us also speaks to Andrena's talent, her near-genius for creating relationships across a myriad of social and cultural border zones. She could create intimacy in all sorts of places. As anthropologists, we may no longer have "research subjects" or even "key informants" in the way we were traditionally taught. But still, for most of us, there is often a wide and deep gulf between us and the people we study and write about. When we make a friend, this is not only a personal gift. It also opens a new kind of window onto the worlds we try to understand. Andrena has been my window. She is the person whose experiences I have returned to again and again in my own reflections while trying to gauge the depth and subtlety of my own depictions. There may be no such thing as authenticity in any romantic sense, but we all know when we have found a way of speaking we judge to be truer, "experience near" enough not to ride roughshod over the events we have witnessed, the people we have come to know. Even when I have not explicitly mentioned Andrena or her daughter Belinda, she has served as a kind of guide in this crucial respect for me.

When I was first introduced to Andrena, she had been suddenly plunged into a terrible dream, as she put it, one that began with the horrifying news that her four-year-old not only had cancer, but cancer of the "worst kind." Upon finding that her daughter has this "worst kind" of brain cancer, Andrena cries out in disbelief, "I'm dreaming, I'm dreaming, I'm dreaming!" Life reverses itself in an instant. What *should* be a nightmare is what is real. Her nightmare set the stage for an earlier book (Mattingly 2010b), and I return to her now to consider the complexities of moral transformation. This parallel play of alternate realities has nowhere been so vividly marked for me than in Andrena's response to her child's illness and her struggle to create a good life, a life worth living.

In what follows I examine how Andrena's unfolding life with her daughter underscores just how her experience compels her to do a kind of experimental learning, a learning to live with diverse and even contradictory storylines—multiple possible futures. This subjunctive mode of attention is not merely passively experienced, and not primarily found in Andrena's storytelling. Rather, it becomes visible through her active efforts to emplot her life and the life of her daughter in such a way that they live out numerous lives at the same time. To illustrate, I offer a series of events that are episodes in this unfolding family story. They reveal how much the sense of living multiple lives and having multiple selves is not simply an individual experience, but one that is interpersonal, and in complicated ways, socially negotiated.

Like the other families in this study, Andrena's situation brings home the social nature of illness and healing. The families themselves could be said to share in the illness. Even the possibility of recovery is a family matter. The parents see themselves as well as their children as sufferers;

it is tremendously difficult and often despairing work to watch over and care for one's very ill or severely disabled child. Andrena's struggle with despair, while contemplating a future in which her child may very well die, has been an intimate and elemental part of the "illness experience" for her. How can she create hope, and how can she see health care as a source of hope? How does she also come to face the possibility that Belinda may die?

She does so both by telling and creating certain sorts of stories about Belinda. She acts in such a way that several plotlines are promoted. She shapes moments with Belinda that further the most hopeful story, the one in which the chemotherapy and radiation and surgery work, the tumor does not grow back, and Belinda gets a chance to grow up. But Andrena and Belinda also participate in other activities that force them to face the darkest story, the one in which Belinda will not live to see another birthday.

I offer some short snippets from their life together that reveal this in a particularly vivid way.

ONE MONTH AFTER DIAGNOSIS: BELINDA HAS SURGERY

With Belinda's illness Andrena faced not only her own fears, but also a sense of her family's betrayal. A few weeks after the diagnosis, Belinda had brain surgery. It was at this point that life changed most dramatically for the whole family. As a result of the surgery, Belinda was suddenly altered. She had to wear a large helmet to protect her head. She was confined to a wheelchair. She lost virtually all of her capabilities. As Andrena put it, "She couldn't walk. She was having trouble even talking and using her hands." She lost a substantial amount of her hearing. She spoke in short, halting sentences, or in the sharply tempered commands of a two-year-old when she spoke at all. Often she seemed lost in a world all her own. Suddenly, the family was faced with a severely disabled little girl. Even in the best scenarios, it was not clear how severe or long-lasting these impairments would be. The dramatic alteration of a bright and talkative child caused unbearable pain for the family. And, as families sometimes do under the press of misery, they fell apart.

Before Belinda's illness, she had lived in a home of six. There were her parents, her adult older sister and her husband, and her nephew—who was a year older than she and as close as any brother. Within months after the diagnosis, their home dissolved. In Andrena's mind, the rest of the family had all "run away," and she found herself in a small apartment with just Belinda. In an early interview she put it this way:

> We were just kinda like sad about my little girl and it seemed like I was the only one willing to accept it. Because now it's only the two of us, my little girl and myself. The other ones, they kind of moved out on me. And they kind of started like picking up a few bad habits [she is speaking especially of Belinda's father, who began an affair with another woman]. And I don't know if they [these bad habits] was already there in the first place or they [her husband] were just waiting for something to happen so they could have an excuse. But, it just seemed like they couldn't take it. Which I couldn't take it either. But, you know, she's my daughter and I thought I was responsible for her. And there was times when I wanted to go in different directions too, but I couldn't. Because I said, "I want to see this thing through with her."

Andrena cannot "go in different directions" but commits to "see[ing] this thing through." And yet, what will she do if her daughter dies? How will she be able to bear it? She confessed, crying, that when she first heard the terrible news, she was struck with such deep despair, she longed to die:

> When I first found out about my daughter I wanted to kill myself. I didn't want to be here if my daughter, if she wasn't going to make it, you know? And I just—and I just kept saying "I don't want to be here."

But this is not the stance she wants to have. Thus, she is confronted by the moral imperative to become a different sort of person, to re-envision her own life so that she can see her daughter differently. She was also struck that she was not *seeing* her daughter in the right way. "I was looking at her, I was already making her gone, you know? Talking like that, I was, just like already making her gone."

She decided she would have to change and she turned to familiar spiritual practices, especially prayer, to help out. As she put it, she "turned it around," referring here not to the course of the disease but to her own stance toward it. She began the difficult work of cultivating hope.

> So I started thinking positive and you know just praying real hard and seeing if she was going to make it. . . . I turned it around and I just kept thinking positive. And that positive kind of prayer, it worked and the hospital was, you know—the people who worked there and everything—they're all doing their parts, you know? So I was just—I was just thanking God. So that's all.

When Andrena concludes here, "So that's all," her single statement belies the complexity of what is involved in learning how to "think positive." It is this complexity, its experimentally that I explore here. "Thinking positive" is no straightforward matter.

SIX MONTHS AFTER DIAGNOSIS: THE I.E.P. MEETING

After Belinda had been through surgery and initial bouts of radiation treatments, she continued with regular intervals of chemotherapy. Despite the initial devastation caused especially by the surgery, things began to improve. Andrena credited Jane, Belinda's favorite physical therapist, with teaching Belinda to walk again. She wobbled and her balance never fully returned, but walk she did. She started talking with more animation, especially to her cousins. Her sense of humor reappeared. Although she continued to fall into a dazed trance-like inertia, she would come to life when something caught her interest.

Andrena began to feel more optimistic. Belinda missed school terribly, but the clinicians advised Andrena that she might be eligible for a special school, equipped for children with disabilities, where she could have some semblance of a normal life. And, if Belinda spent time in school, Andrena speculated, perhaps she herself could go back to school as well. Everything had changed now anyway. She'd lost her job of eleven years because she had missed so much work caring for Belinda. As she watched Belinda regain some of her strength, she reconsidered her life. Perhaps this loss could open a few new doors. She might change careers. She had been a receptionist for a car dealership, pleasant but not especially rewarding work. This could be a chance for real change, for a job that had more purpose. She could train to be a nurse, or at least a nurse's aide. After all, she surmised, she had already had months of learning about clinical work as part of caring for her daughter, including acquiring some technical skills. She was now adept at doing physical and occupational therapy home exercises with Belinda, reading x-rays and tracking side effects to medicines based on experience and Internet research. She had even become expert at giving shots, since she administered chemotherapy to Belinda at home. Beyond these newly acquired technical competencies, Andrena now had a wealth of experience about how to ease a child's pain or how to comfort fellow parents she had met in the hospital as they anguished over their child's illnesses. She had gained a new network of friends—other parents she met in clinic waiting rooms, or parents of children Belinda befriended during her many in-patient stays in the hospital. She learned a great deal from their experiences as well.

Andrena made up her mind to do something. She searched neighboring areas near her house and finally found a school she hoped might take Belinda. She spoke to school staff and they set up an I.E.P.

(Individualized Education Plan) to evaluate Belinda and determine whether she would be an appropriate candidate. They were especially concerned with whether she had the required cognitive and speech skills. They also wanted to examine her motor deficits, which might entail special safety measures. Andrena asked me to come along to the meeting, which I did.

We met in an empty classroom with a committee of three, including a special education teacher, a speech therapist, and the school psychologist, who took charge. Andrena introduced me as her sister. The school professionals looked startled, but they nodded. The psychologist gave Belinda some small tests to do, while the rest of us waited. Belinda seemed especially alert that day, and she tried hard. Andrena discussed Belinda's medical condition with the three of them, including where she was currently receiving treatment. A half-hour later, they showed us to the door and told Andrena they would get in touch with her after they ascertained whether they had open spots in an appropriate classroom. "Belinda really misses school," Andrena told them pleadingly. "She just loves children and she hates being home by herself all the time. She needs to learn!" The psychologist nodded, smiling but impossible to read. I had no idea whether they would admit Belinda or not, but Andrena was optimistic as I walked her and Belinda back to her car down the block. "This would be so great for her," she confided. "And did you see their faces when I said you were my sister?" She grinned. "They didn't know what to think!" We laughed. "But you know," she added, "they'll take me more seriously with you there. Or anyway, they might." I gave her a hug and headed to my own car.

Andrena got a call a week later. The school might be able to take Belinda but because it was already April, they decided it was too late for that school year. They vaguely suggested that perhaps there would be a summer school program she could attend. They also told Andrena they would need further documentation from the oncologist that Belinda was truly well enough to be in school. September was a long way off, and Andrena was quite disappointed at their decision.

SEVEN MONTHS AFTER DIAGNOSIS: BELINDA'S FIFTH BIRTHDAY PARTY AT CHUCK E. CHEESE

In late March, Belinda turned five. Andrena planned a big party at a local Chuck E. Cheese. Belinda had been begging for this party for weeks and Andrena, who just heard the devastating news that the MRI showed new cancerous growth in her brain, decided to move the party up one week before they started massive chemotherapy again. She invited several of us on the research team and asked us to videotape, which we did. If you have never visited such a place, you just have to imagine an amusement park and a pizza place crammed into one very cavernous indoor room, filled to the brim with yelling kids playing all kinds of games while harassed parents try to keep up with them or slump at nearby tables drinking Coke and eating slices of pizza.

When we got there, Belinda looked tired and thin. She was mostly bald and her steps were wobbly, but she was dressed in her favorite Pocahontas outfit and she trooped off to play every possible game with her cousins. Sometimes she looked more like a soldier on a march than a five-year-old girl at her own party. She seemed relentlessly determined to enjoy herself. She moved among a large circle of friends and family members. Even Andrena's sister, who didn't get along well with Andrena, had come with her children.

Andrena seemed just as determined as Belinda to eke pleasure from this party. She stepped in and encouraged Belinda whenever she wavered or became overwhelmed or dazed. There were moments when Belinda became tense and uncertain. At such times, Andrena and other family members moved in quickly to ease her along as though collectively orchestrating Belinda's experience. A moment early in the party illustrates this.

Belinda approached a (stationary) motorcycle ride—interested but tentative, shying away from other children near the ride. Her aunt helped her onto one of the motorcycles. When it started to move, she held the bars tightly, looking straight ahead, unsmiling. As soon as the ride finished, Andrena took her to a mechanical horse ride. As she was helping her up a young girl approached, asking if Belinda was getting off. Andrena replied in cheery determination, "Nope, she's getting *on*." Andrena called out to Belinda in cheerleader fashion as the horse started to move: "C'mon Belinda! Look at Belinda!" Belinda, struggling with her balance and alternately watching other children play, nervously clutched the reins as she tried to stay on. It was only after much coaching and cheering that Belinda visibly relaxed. Having mastered motorcycle and horse, Belinda grew bolder, even jostling aside other children to get her turn at a ball toss or another ride. Andrena drew back, smiling as she watched Belinda play.

One of the remarkable features of this event was Andrena's apparent carelessness with Belinda. She allowed her to wander off with other children who had come to the party, or at times even let Belinda go off by herself. I could see Belinda making her unsteady way among clamorous groups of children. Once she was pushed hard by a child and knocked down by another. She even got in trouble. She walked off with a ball belonging to one of the games that she refused to give up until a security guard came over to take it from her. Andrena watched this from afar, doing nothing to stop her.

I had never seen Andrena careless with Belinda. So what was this about? She seemed to have her own fierce desire to give Belinda this party in a way that *enacted* a normal child's party. And in fact, as the party progressed, Belinda shifted from a scared child, afraid to play with other children, fearful of the games and dazed, to a willful child who *wanted* things and was willing to get in trouble or cause trouble to get them. It was likely a sign of her sickness that she was allowed to get into such trouble. (Andrena never let her grandson or other children in the family be ill mannered in public.) But, trouble is also part of children's everyday lives. Here, as much as anywhere, Andrena showed a stubborn insistence on giving her daughter a real birthday party, one that came with the squabbles of child's play.

Narratively, what kind of event is this party? Is it a milestone in a bright future, the fifth of many more birthdays? Or is it a kind of last supper, the final party? Both meanings seem to be present at the same time.

FOURTEEN MONTHS AFTER DIAGNOSIS: BELINDA RETURNS TO SCHOOL

It took several more months before Andrena was able to find a school that would take Belinda, one where Andrena felt "safe" to leave her daughter. Fourteen months after diagnosis, Belinda finally returned to school. Andrena described Belinda's first day at school (in mid-December) as well as Andrena's own relief and delight at this occasion. Andrena recounted standing in the classroom doorway watching the teacher try to get Belinda to put her backpack away and sit down with the other children. Laughingly, Andrena described some tussling between the teacher and Belinda, who wanted to "take off" and run around the classroom.

> When I took her yesterday, I was trying to see what all really went on in her class. The teacher had to call her back to the front because she got in that classroom and she took off. And then, the teacher had to show her where her little slot was to put her backpack. So, she came back and she put—the

teacher explained to her—and she put it up real quick and she took off again. And then I was just standing there, like, I don't know, waiting to see if she was going to like, make a run out of the building or what.

Finally, the teacher settled her down. A mixture of relief *and* sadness suddenly struck Andrena.

I was just, like, just kept standing there at the door to see if she was going to have any reactions. . . . "Belinda" [she called to her]. And then I said to myself, "You're not supposed to be hollering in class." And she turned around and then she just, like, turned her head back around. The teacher told me, "You act like you want to cry instead of Belinda." But I was just in shock.

In this story, she described herself *still* in the doorway, calling out her daughter's name. But once again Belinda is surrounded by other school-children and simply ignores her mother. Andrena laughingly chided her-self for calling out to her daughter in school. "You're not supposed to be hollering in class!" She continued this self-mocking narrative by describing Belinda's internal dialogue. Smiling, Andrena imagined Belin-da's annoyance: "What you still standing there for? Get out!"

Andrena offers a classic "first day of school" tale, a humorous reversal in which it is the parent rather than the child who suffers from separation anxiety. This little tale symbolically places Belinda back into the "normal" world of children where the biggest drama concerns leav-ing home. A few seconds later, Andrena underscores this point when she sums up what school means for both of them. It signals a beginning in an unfolding narrative of return and recovery.

I'm glad she's having a chance to get out there and just start in with her little life. And it would be, like, you know, a big break for me. It's like four hours. But that's a start. And [she adds ironically] I can find something to do. Four hours!

Belinda's new school is a special education facility for children with disabilities rather than the "regular ed" preschool Belinda once attended. Andrena reiterates several times that this school has two nurses who are "real nurses," not "nurse assistants." She felt reassured by the many detailed questions they asked her about Belinda's immune system. She thought she was leaving her child in the hands of real professionals. Andrena noted some friends and families were critical of her for putting her daughter in a special needs classroom. But she did not agree with them. She gives us a glimpse of the internal ethical dialogue that accom-panies decisions like this one.

They were saying, "Oh, I wouldn't let my daughter go to a school where it's all handicapped kids and everything because she might start, you know, regressing or whatever." But again, I didn't listen to them. I went to the school myself and I saw how they take the time with the kids and everything, and how they teach them and how they watch them, you know, closely. That's my main concern. Instead of taking her to a regular school, where kids would be running over her and pushing her down, knocking her upside the head. I mean, like, bumping her which would hit her head and everything. And I said [to myself], "I don't care what they say. I'm taking her where she gets what's good for her. Later on, you know, when things change . . . or whatever, she could go to a regular school. But right now, this is what she needs and this is what I need, and I'm happy."

When Andrena says "later on" her daughter might go to "regular school," she reveals how deeply she is invested in a future story in which recovery is a genuine possibility.

ELEVEN MONTHS AFTER DIAGNOSIS: A PARALLEL PLOT—BEFRIENDING DREA AT THE COLLECTIVE NARRATIVE GROUP

I have begun to sketch one kind of plot with certain key moments that unfolded since Belinda's diagnosis. I have offered moments of Andrena's and Belinda's life that figure as episodes in an arduous yet promising healing journey. There is the terrifying diagnosis, Andrena's shock and depression and the disintegration of the family. But then there is an answer from Andrena: her determination to re-envision her life and her future in a narrative of hope, of possibility. Whatever else, she declares, her daughter was not "already gone," and she seems to have refused to allow herself that future story. She prays for strength to reimagine her future in this more hopeful way, to be with her child on this journey, wherever it may take them. And she takes practical steps with some success, giving her child a big birthday party, even finding a school willing to take Belinda, one with "real nurses" who will keep her child safe. There follows the "miracle" of a first day-at-school experience, a quintessential beginning story in a "normal" child's life; miraculous in its very mundane-ness—a drama of ordinary life. This moment of ordinariness marks the highest hope—this is "an experience" in an anticipated story of return, a light that momentarily promises a way out of the darkness and despair that cancer has brought to this family.

I now backtrack a few months to introduce another plotline that also runs through Andrena's life during this period. In the midst of this journey that seems to promise healing and even some return to normalcy,

Andrena does something puzzling. She befriends Drea, another mother in the study. Drea's child is near death. This child's diagnosis and even her oncologist are the same as Belinda's. What is so surprising about Andrena's actions is that Drea is vocal about giving up on herself as well as her child's recovery. Drea is drowning in her own sorrow and despair. Andrena repeatedly told me she had refused to see some of her friends who thought she should "just let Belinda go." Though it might seem that Andrena insists upon a simple optimism, this is belied by her simultaneous efforts to face an opposing future story, creating experiences and taking actions that compel her to recognize a much darker possibility.

Andrena and Drea met at a family group meeting we had organized as part of the research. In chapter 4, I briefly described these collective narrative groups when one of them was the setting for Delores's dog food story. Andrena had been part of the collective narratives from the very beginning. Drea joined several months later, in October 1998. Andrena quickly found out that Drea's daughter Sashi was only a year older than Belinda, and she, too, had been diagnosed—also at four and a half—with the exact type of brain cancer that Belinda had. However, the progress of Sashi's cancer was much swifter than Belinda's. By the time of this meeting in October 1998, Sashi was on a ventilator at home because Drea had fought to get her daughter out of the hospital.

I recount a conversation among the parents, including Andrena, that occurred as Drea introduced herself to the group and told a story about her child's cancer. Drea mentioned how critically ill her daughter was now. With a flat voice, Drea added that her daughter's oncologist was going to discuss the case with a colleague at another renowned clinic to see if some kind of experimental chemotherapy might reverse the cancer. Listening intently to this, Andrena remarked, "There's still hope." Drea said nothing, a potent silence. Another mother concurred with Andrena and Andrena repeated, "There's still hope, and she's still here." Yet another mother added a story about a cousin of hers who the doctors predicted would die by the time he was five. Now he was thirty-one. He could not walk or move, but still he was alive. This mother concluded, "So you can't say what a person can't do. You know? And she [the mother], she held on for her son."

In response to all this, Drea continued to say nothing. She cried silently, her face impassive. When someone asked if Sashi was her only child, she finally spoke. Her words were stark. "It's my baby. She's five. They gave her two months to live."

Andrena responded immediately, telling a story of her own despair and struggle for hope. In fact she described her struggle with despair in terms more direct than she had ever used before in this family group. As she talked, she leaned to face Drea while speaking. It was as though the rest of us were not even there:

> Well, the grateful part is, there's still the time for you to feel like [she wavers, her voice shaking, and then goes on] God, you know, 'cause I was feeling like [pausing, taking a deep breath]. When I first found out, when they was telling me, "Oh, she might not make it," I was saying, "but if she don't make it, I'm gonna kill myself." I was just thinking like that, you know? And I know I meant it. I'm sure I meant it. But I have a better outlook on it now. But I was saying that at first . . . I was feeling like that. I was sayin' "If something happens to her, it's gonna do it to me too." But, I just keep giving hope and I keep giving prayers, you know? Because they've been working. I know that the doctors, they do whatever they do and I know and, from my own feelings, I know God is doing his part too. So, I just, I still pray 'cause I know it's really not over yet. [she adds, softly] Each day that she has is more time, you know?

Here, Andrena concluded by offering Drea the coda: "Each day she has hope. Each day." When another mother (one whose child was not suffering from a life-threatening illness) jumped in and said to Drea, "She could wake up and just be totally healed. Don't let no doctor tell me that my child couldn't make it!" Andrena quickly intervened. Still facing Drea, she commented, "But it's painful. I know. It's painful because that's natural. It's painful hearing what they [the clinicians] have to say." A few minutes later, the conversation turned again to Drea. Andrena was startled to discover that their children had the same oncologist, Dr. Hilger.

Andrena: What's her [your daughter's] name?

Drea: Sashi.

Andrena: Sashi. Who's her doctor?

Drea: Um, Dr. Hilger.

Andrena: (Smiles, confidently. She trusts Dr. Hilger.) Oh, she gonna be here forever.

(All laugh)

Drea: (Shaking her head) No, because he's like, giving up too.

Andrena: (Frowns in surprise) Really?

Andrena is disconcerted that the physician she has come to trust has "given up" on Drea's daughter. She becomes even more disconcerted to find out that Sashi was diagnosed even later than Belinda and is so much sicker.

Andrena: How long has she had it?

Drea: Um, she was diagnosed in December.

Andrena: Oh, just last year?

Drea: Mm-hmm.

Andrena: Oh.

Another mother: So it came on pretty quick, huh?

Andrena and Drea exchanged phone numbers at the end of the meeting and Andrena began to call Drea at home. She spoke of Drea often when I saw her, mentioning her visits to Drea's house where she and Belinda would frequently visit Sashi. "Drea needs cheering up," Andrena would tell me. "She's feeling very down. She feels like she's all alone." Strikingly, Andrena stayed close to Drea and her daughter right through the end.

Here is Andrena, looking straight in the face of the darkest story, and also perhaps letting Belinda glimpse that possible terrible future—though she never talked to me about it in this way. The possible future that Andrena looks at not only concerns her own daughter's likely death but her own potential to become suicidal in the face of its immanent likelihood. Drea viscerally embodied the loss of hope. This can be heard in the story she shares with us the day after a doctor tells her that Sashi has only one year to live. Drea noted that at first she was not too worried.

> You know when they told me that it was a tumor, I was like, oh okay and go ahead and get it and then everything will be all right. [But the following news devastates her] The doctor said to me yesterday afterwards the diagnosis is like a year [to live]. [She shakes her head here at how this news is delivered] Dr. Mandrake, I mean he is not a bad person. I like him. But for him to call me in there and tell me that my child is going to d-i-e [spells it]. I was like, wow. And then he is asking, "How's the sister doing? Do you have any guns in the house? Anyone suicidal? Do you think you would resort to drugs and alcohol and stuff'?" I just straight told him, "I don't know. Because I don't know what the future holds. And I don't know how it might affect me." And he said, "Oh, is this a problem that you have?" [She remarks bitterly] "No, it's not a problem that I have. But I just can't say 'no' 'cause you never know what may happen. I hope not, you know, but you never know what may happen."

Drea struggled to find hope, but after this discussion with the doctor, and as her daughter got sicker, she could no longer embrace the idea that her daughter might live. She did not—as Andrena did—cultivate any image of a "miracle" healing. Rather, she spoke of simply enduring the pain, of a stoic acceptance and the chance of a vague future blessing from God once she has "taken the blows" that cancer has brought. This was all she could hope for.

> I just go through and what happens [is] I just accept it and just keep going. Because there is nothing, what else can I do? If I break down and if I fall apart that's not going to do me no good. So I have to just, you know, keep taking the blows, you know, and get on up. Because you know what? All the blows aren't going to keep knocking me down. That's what I was just thinking at the laundromat. I said 'When God is going to bless and when He blesses it going to be something else.' But you know, I probably just have to go through this first. So I'm just going through it. You see these people talking all the time about trial and tribulations. I know just what they talking about.

When Sashi fell into a coma at home, Andrena not only visited her, but took Belinda on one of her visits. Andrena recounted how Belinda had climbed into the bed with Sashi, put her arms around her, and just lay down beside her.

THIRTEEN MONTHS AFTER DIAGNOSIS: SASHI DIES AND DREA CONFRONTS PARENTS WHO HOPE

Two months after the collective narrative where Andrena met Drea, Drea's daughter died. Andrena went to Sashi's funeral, though she didn't take Belinda this time. Andrena was so distraught that she barely recognized people she knew there. And yet she let herself experience this event. Perhaps even more remarkably, she tried to stay close to Drea after Sashi's death, although Drea held out no hope that Belinda would live.

After her daughter's death, Drea became increasingly angry. I offer a bit of a heated exchange that ensued with other parents at the last of the collective narrative groups she ever attended. It began when parents (father Andrew and mother Darlene), whose daughter Arlene was also critically ill (and would die a few months later), described their daughter's dire situation. They told Drea they understood how it might feel to lose a child. To this Drea furiously retorted they could not possibly know. She also obliquely suggested that keeping a critically ill child "alive" (that is, keeping her heart and vital organs going) when she was "brain dead" (the choice Andrew and Darlene had made) was morally wrong. Drea emerges as the one parent in the family group who was willing, even relieved, to "let her [Sashi] go" at this final stage. She followed medical advice to not resuscitate her daughter, advice some other families in the group had refused to take. But in aligning herself with what the clinicians advised, Drea was aware that she might seem callous, uncaring, or lacking sufficient strength to keep hoping and fighting for her daughter. This could be heard in the way Andrew and Darlene, two of the parents whose situation is considered in the following chapter, and Drea talk to one another in the following snippet of conversation.

Darlene described her child's many resuscitations in the NICU. Andrena said nothing during the exchange. She only listened attentively, tearfully.

> *Darlene:* At the first of the year, her [child's] chest was burned up too from all the stimulating there and rubbing, the skin had burnt off. And all we— we'd been there—they told us that she was going to be a vegetable, she would never move or nothing. I told them I was going to be her guardian. I can't. I can't [let her go].
>
> *Drea:* I just did not like that anymore. To see my baby just burnt up like that, with nothing up here. And she arrested seven times. I mean, how many people do you know, grown people, that have seven heart attacks and survive? But once they got her going, they put her on three heart medicines. She just laid up there. You know, nothing. So it's like, just let her go. We had the pastor come in and, you know—(sighs, trailing off).
>
> *Darlene:* So when she was, when she passed, she was still on the heart medicine?
>
> *Drea:* Yeah, but she was dead. But they just had the heart medicine going. You know? They had did CAT scans and all that. She was dead. You know? So it just didn't make no sense. I mean, to just lay up there dead and have heart medicine going. She's just going to lay up there forever like that? With heart medicine? It didn't make no sense. I had to kind of, you know, put my feelings aside and kind of look at that thing. You know, she wasn't going to come back from that.
>
> *Darlene:* Oh, see Arlene [her critically ill daughter] still has movement and [she] still look around and be touched.
>
> *Drea:* Yeah. And I agree. I agree. I would have did the same thing. And I did the same thing all the way up until the end, but you know, it was just that time. You know? But I knew it was coming, so I just had to, you know, face it. You know?
>
> *Darlene:* Yeah. And we—
>
> *Drea:* (Interrupts) I know that she don't have to suffer no more. I'm glad I don't have to deal with those wishy-washy-ass doctors, nurses, you know. All those people. It's like a big burden released off of me. You know, I really, I feel a lot better. Now, I miss her. You know? And no one could ever replace her, but I just, I'm sure she feels better. (Voice lowers, tremulous) She's resting. I feel better. It's just, we're going on with our lives. It's

just a lot different. Oh, we miss her. Don't get me wrong. It's just that time. They gave me a year to prepare myself for it, but the time came and I still wasn't prepared. You know? (Silent tears now run down her face.) You go and you see your baby in the hospital, and then the next time you see her, she's laying in a casket.

Darlene: (sighing) Shew! I—I can relate—

Drea: (fiercely) Hm-mm. No, you can't. No, you can't.

Darlene: Oh, yes I can.

Drea: (voice rising) No, you can't. Not unless you've been there and done that.

Darlene: No, no, no, no, no, no.

Drea: Then you can't relate.

Darlene: No, I can relate to just seeing Arlene paralyzed and—

Drea: She's still got life—

Darlene: —was still in a coma, wasn't moving, wasn't doing nothing—

Drea: She's still got life.

Darlene: Ooh!

Drea: You—you—that's the end of the rope. When you go to the mortuary. You know, that's it and that's all.

Darlene: (listening) Yeah.

Drea: And when you—you—when you deal with that, then you talk to me about it. When you—nu-uh, you ain't dealing with that. It's like a—wooh! Science fiction movie, like just . . . like, where am I? What is happening? You know?

Darlene: (silently nods) Mm-hmm.

Drea: And you still trying to keep a grip. You know, you're still trying to hold it all in. That's just something else. I mean, it gets you, 'Cause I love, I love my children. You know. I put them before I put myself. So (pauses) nothing is harder than that. You can bury your momma, you can bury daddy, your sister, and your brother. But when you bury your child . . . (softly) hm-mm. That's something I wouldn't wish on my worst enemy. To have to bury your child. (pauses) But we hanging though. We coming through. I used to always say that, too. Like, nobody never really died close to me—never—knock on wood (knocks on table). And then I was faced with it. (sighing) It's over now. (pause) (softly) I tell you—it's . . . it's just like it turns the world upside down.

Drea's agony was palpable. She declared herself tired of the "wishy-washy-ass" doctors and nurses. It was better that her daughter was dead, although this too was unbearable. The utter bleakness of her words was matched by the language of her body. She cried, clenching her fists, angry at the room. She asked everyone what good it was to come to this group anymore. "Am I a benefit to it if I am a burden?" Others rushed to reassure her they wanted her to return. Andrena's quiet response revealed her own sense of kinship with Drea. "If you don't come, I won't have a partner." Though turning specifically to Andrena, Drea tells the group she is pregnant with another child. Parents congratulate her and, as can be seen in the following exchange, she asks Andrena to come with her to the doctor.

Darlene: Congratulations on your new baby.

Drea: Thank you.

Darlene: Congratulations on that.

Andrena: Congratulations to you too.

Drea: I got to go to the doctor; you want to go with me?

Andrena: (nodding enthusiastically) Girl! (Others laugh.)

Despite the solidarity Andrena expressed to Drea during this meeting, it was clear from many subsequent interviews that she struggled with Drea's position. Drea confronted her in two fundamental ways. She rejected the possibility of a miracle cure for her own child. This is a rejection of a subjunctive stance that Andrena (like most of the parents in our study) insisted on holding. Drea also disturbed Andrena because of her negative view of the clinicians, many of them the very same ones treating Belinda. Drea told Andrena they had basically "forgotten" Sashi when they determined there was nothing more they could do medically. Like one of Marley's ghosts, Drea points a finger at Andrena's most dreaded future, one where she and her daughter are abandoned and her daughter is left to die. As Belinda got sicker, Andrena mulled over Drea's portrait of the hospital staff.

I don't know why Drea said like "When they [the clinicians] think that it's nothing they can do, they just stop acting like your child is important." . . . She said that they did that with Sashi. She said that at the end, the doctors didn't even, sometimes, didn't want to look at her or whatever when she brought Sashi for her little appointments and things.

A few months after her daughter's death, Drea "disappeared." When Andrena wanted to send Drea a card in remembrance of Sashi's birthday, she could no longer get hold of her. Her phone had been disconnected. Andrena speculated that Drea had quite literally disconnected from Andrena partly because Andrena still saw hope for her own daughter's recovery and Drea saw her "in denial." Andrena said:

> Then all of a sudden she just stopped talking. When she first started talking about Belinda . . . it was already going to be over with. [In Drea's mind] And I said, "she still has a chance" and everything like that. So she probably thought I was like in denial or something, you know? But she said "well when the time comes, then I'll share with you, about what I went through."

As it turned out, Andrena guesses correctly here. Drea did believe that Belinda would also die, and she feared that Andrena "will not be able to take it" when this happened. Drea once remarked when she was still in contact with Andrena:

> I don't wanna say this and I hope Belinda survives, but I don't think she's gonna survive. I just don't think she's gonna make it. And I just know I have to be there for Andrena. I hope she makes it. But I just don't think Andrena will be able to take it. She's sensitive.

Drea's certainty about Belinda's probable death made Andrena's attempt to create a close friendship with her so powerful. It speaks to the complexity of Andrena's practice of hope and to work of moral transformation this involved. Not only did Andrena go to visit Drea when her daughter was in a coma, she tried to stay close after Sashi's death, knowing that Drea envisioned Belinda's imminent death. Beyond this, Drea's hopelessness about her own life once her daughter died enacted Andrena's most fearful future of all—the one Andrena was desperate to avoid, where she herself would not have the "strength" to go on if Belinda died.

EIGHTEEN MONTHS AFTER DIAGNOSIS: BELINDA DIES

Belinda fell into a coma two weeks before she died. Andrena had her at home with hospice nurses coming to help give care. Her house was crowded with family members and friends. Whenever I went to visit, I would find Belinda lying on the large double bed (that she and Andrena shared) while cousins lay beside her, watching TV. Andrena thought Belinda might still be able to hear so she kept children's shows on continually. Since Belinda loved to play with her cousins, Andrena was happy to have them with her on the bed. Other cousins and family members piled into the living room. Suddenly Andrena's family world was full. Andrena had mixed feelings about all this company. "Sometimes I wish they'd all leave so I could just be with my Belinda by myself," she confessed to me. She enjoyed the children, who cuddled Belinda and jostled with one another on the bed. But some of the adults, especially her ex-husband's mother and sisters, irritated her to no end. They were full of advice. But Andrena felt she had been dealing with this for so long that their show of support often irked rather than comforted her. She pulled me aside to complain about this on my visits.

Finally Andrena did send everyone away. Belinda died in her arms one night, only two weeks after she had slipped into this final coma. Andrena heard her very last heartbeat. Belinda was ten days shy of her sixth birthday.

FIVE DAYS LATER: BELINDA'S FUNERAL

The funeral took place a few days after her death. I had already been to several funerals in Andrena's family, although I had only known Andrena for a year and a half. There was Andrena's mother who died of stomach cancer. Her older sister (just forty-five) died of kidney failure. Her ex-husband, father to her one other child (Belinda's older sister) had also died, though only in his mid-forties. She was devastated by the losses of her sister and especially her mother, to whom she was very close. Her own father had died a few months before Belinda was diagnosed. This relentless onslaught of family deaths shattered Andrena. She told me over and over that she couldn't see how she could have the strength to face Belinda's death without even her mother there. Belinda and her grandmother, both undergoing chemotherapy, had often traded scarves to cover their bare heads. Over a two-year period, Andrena was not only steeped in death, it seemed to her that she was burying her family by herself. Her mother's burial was especially lonely because her one sister had already passed away and her only brother was in prison. He tried but could not get permission for a release to attend the service.

Belinda's funeral was different. It was clear that Andrena had been planning this a long time, as I discovered when I arrived for the service. My first surprise was the memorial's location. It was not in the Inglewood cemetery where her mother, father, and sister lay. Belinda's funeral was to take place far away from Andrena's neighborhood in South Central LA, to the northeast of the city, near Universal Studios and Studio City, the home of so many Hollywood movies. Mary Lawlor and I drove together. As we approached this part of LA, we were dismayed to see how "disembodied" it looked, gigantic buildings and huge parking lots manned by guards. Who would want to be buried in a place near this? I wondered. We rechecked the address as we sped by lot after empty lot lined with movie trailers and an enormous expanse of gray buildings. It was a world of concrete.

We finally found the cemetery. We stopped at a gate with an information booth. The cemetery grounds themselves consisted of rolling green hills with a few clumps of trees. The lawns looked eerily manicured, well watered like a golf course. I couldn't place what was wrong until we noticed that there were no standing gravestones, just flat white squares in the closely trimmed grass. Hundreds of graves punched into a green expanse—so many uniform blank spaces. There was no little church like the one Andrena regularly attended near her house, or where her other family members had their memorial services. Instead, the service was to be held inside a large, square, impersonal pseudo-colonial building, all white with gold gilding.

We went inside the chapel and sat down. Already there were several dozen people sitting in the pews. We read the printed programs we had been given. They too were startling. A picture of Belinda covered the front of the program. She looked a bit wan and thin, but she was in a pretty party dress. Above her photo were the words "Happy Birthday Belinda!" The same picture and caption were also on a large poster placed in the front of the chapel so that we could see it immediately upon entering the doorway. Obviously, Andrena had decided (being sure this is what Belinda would want) to make this a last birthday party for her. And as Andrena later put it, it was also a "going-away party." The inside of the program was filled with pictures of Belinda—Belinda sick, Belinda in a coma, Belinda before she had cancer, Belinda through every age of her short life.

A few minutes later Andrena entered, dressed all in blue (Belinda's favorite color). She sat up front. The pews were now completely full. The background music played softly. I looked up at the ceiling. It was painted like a stage set starry night, dark blue splashed with gold twinkling stars. Andrena's pastor walked on to the stage, and when the service itself started, the Hollywood ambience disappeared. Things became very real. Andrena's pastor presided over the ceremony. In Reverend Black's opening, he asked people to treat this as a "celebration." The message of strength filled the pastor's initial prayer:

> We thank you Lord God for your grace and for your mercy. We pray right now that you would touch each and every family member, each and every friend, each and every individual that is in this room today, that you would

bless them with your sweet comfort, with your strength and your power. We pray particularly for the family Lord, that you would strengthen them. Strengthen mom, strengthen dad, and grandparents, and godparents, and cousins, uncles and aunts.

The first solo, sung by a young man in a clear alto voice, tellingly spoke of suffering as a path to righteousness.

> I'm learning how to live holy
> and I'm learning how to live right.
> I'm learning, I'm learning
> How to suffer.
> For if I suffer
> I will gain eternal life.

This chorus, repeated several times, promises that at the end of this road of learning how to suffer there will be release.

> For when I see Jesus.
> Amen.
> When I see the man who died for me
> The man that set me free.
> Amen.
> All my heartaches
> All my troubles will be over.

A prerecorded song followed the solo. The pastor told us it was called "Am I Dreaming?" I was reminded of my first interview with Andrena, when she told me that she felt like she was "dreaming" upon hearing the news of her child's cancer. I was evidently not the only one haunted by the dreamlike quality of her images of suffering. This surrealistic mood, a kind of twilight of the mind, was obviously powerfully marked by Andrena as well as evidenced by the song she chose to play. Here are the lyrics.

> Things are kind of hazy
> And my head's all cloudy inside
> And I've heard talk of angels
> I never thought I'd have one to call mine.
>
> See you are
> Just too good to be true
> And I hope
> This is not some kind of mirage with you.
>
> Am I dreaming?
> Am I just imagining you're here in my life?

Am I dreaming?
Pinch me to see if it's real, 'cause my mind can't decide.

Will this last for one night
Or do I have you for a lifetime?
Please say that it's forever
And that it's not an illusion to my eyes.

And I hope
That you don't run out and disappear.
My love, I pray
That it's not a hoax and it's for real.
Am I dreaming?
Am I just imagining you're here in my life?
Am I dreaming?
Pinch me to see if it's real 'cause my mind can't decide.

Sometimes, sometimes
I need you to show me, show me that it's not a mirage.
I need you, I need you, I need you to pinch me
Pinch me to see if it's real 'cause my mind can't decide.

Am I dreaming?
Am I just imagining you're here in my life?
Am I dreaming?
Pinch me to see if it's real 'cause my mind can't decide.

Am I dreaming?
Am I just imagining you're here in my life?
Am I dreaming?

When the song was over, Reverend Black opened the service to remarks from the audience. One by one, people came up to the pulpit to talk about Belinda. They talked from the heart, telling story after story, often speaking directly to Andrena. Few had notes. This testifying, so familiar now, remade the blank strangeness of a stage-set funeral home. It became a different space, weighted, the air palpable with sorrow. There were stories of a family's everyday life. I could have been back in Andrena's church, not in this odd world, next door to major Hollywood studios.

To my great surprise, after several people had spoken, Andrena walked up to the podium. She had never spoken at any of the other funerals of her family I had attended. At her sister's, she was so distraught she had more or less collapsed in the pew while family members put their arms around her. She had refused even to go up to the casket as everyone else was doing. But for this service, Andrena was composed. She did not cry. And when she stood to speak to us, she spoke firmly, her tone passionate but clear. Here is what she said:

Andrena: I want to thank everybody, everybody who was a part of my daughter's life. And I am so grateful that my daughter (pausing to keep herself from weeping), I'm, I'm gonna miss her. Oh, God knows I'm gonna miss her. But, she's never gonna leave me.

Audience: Amen.

Andrena: That little girl, she, she fought so hard for so long, you know. She had an excellent doctor, Dr. Hilger. He told me everything, you know. I mean everything fell into place. . . . He was honest with me about everything. And—hospital, they did a, they did a lovely job. Just wasn't their call. It was God's call. And I'm so grateful that my baby's in heaven, 'cause I know she's there right now.

Audience: Amen.

Andrena: I have no regrets. You know, 'cause she did everything she needed to do, and everything she wanted to do in her whole lifetime.

Audience: Amen.

Andrena: No regrets. Help me bless, you know, 'cause she did everything she needed to do, and everything she wanted to do in her whole lifetime, you know. She did everything, everything she wanted, she had. Everything she needed she had. She had love.

Audience: Amen.

Andrena: And Jesus has given me strength.

Audience: Amen.

Andrena: To take, to take, to take each blessing. And Belinda (she pauses to gather herself). Because I asked Jesus at the end, when my baby, when she could not go on anymore. I told her that it was okay to go on. And I told her I would do everything possible, and God willing, I would be with her again. I asked Jesus at the end, I said to him, "Right here. Take her Jesus. Take her, and heal her with you." And I know she's healed. You guys, you know what? This is, this is not a sad [thing], you know? Because Belinda, Belinda is happy all the time. I used to just stare at her. I used to just stare at her. And I look at her, and she catch me looking at her, and she said, what you looking at me for?

(Laughter and nods of recognition)

Andrena: Belinda, she used to take her time, you know. She, she kissed me in each eye and then I clap. And then she know that I love her more and I wanted more so she kissed me again. And she'd always tell that it'd be alright. She'd always, she'd always come and tell me "It's gonna be alright." You know, that's why I'm taking her word, and Jesus word and I know it's gonna be alright. And, Belinda will be six in a few days, you know. And it would be her, her birthday. And she's still havin' her birthday. Her life is going on in heaven forever. She probably out there now, with us in this room. And if you guys want to see her again, just follow Jesus.

Audience: Amen.

Andrena: And you guys will see her again. I promise you guys you'll see her again.

Audience: Amen.

Andrena: Okay, I love you guys.

Andrena's poignant funeral speech announced that healing was not only related to what God could offer, but what she and the health professionals could offer. Healing meant that each of them, in their own way, gave whatever they could to help Belinda stay alive and be as happy and fulfilled as possible while she lived. For Andrena, it meant that she could say "I have no regrets" because her daughter "did everything she needed to do, and everything she wanted to do, in her whole lifetime." Even if that short lifetime was just a week shy of her sixth birthday. This included getting the best medical care she could for her daughter and finding an "excellent doctor," one who "told me everything" and who made sure that "everything fell into place." As things turned out, healing took place in another space and by other hands, for Belinda was "healed in heaven."

Andrena sat down and there was another song. The notes hung in the air. A final prayer was given by the reverend. We then filed out of the little chapel to the gravesite where Belinda's coffin was to be lowered into the ground. Above the gravesite stood two giant clouds of blue balloons, fifteen feet high and two shades of blue. They floated, tethered above us. I looked down and saw that I was standing on a tombstone and it was also a child's grave. We discovered that all the graves around us were of children. This was, in fact, a child's graveyard. The children who came to the funeral were everywhere as well. They crowded round the open grave and ran through the grass. Several of them passed out balloons among the adults until we each had one.

As the casket was lowered in the ground, we stood with our balloons and sang "Happy Birthday" to Belinda. Andrena told us to let our balloons go. They ascended—a blue cloud against a blue sky. At that same moment, Belinda was lowered into the ground, buried with her favorite purse. Andrena stood by the grave. She told us she could just see her there, glad she could get her purse with "no one to fuss at her," ready to find some other children to play with. And then I realized why Andrena was burying her here, far away from the rest of her family. Belinda needed a childhood still. Knowing Belinda was a very social girl, Andrena wanted to make sure she wasn't lonely, that she was surrounded with playmates. You could see the playfulness marked by the many children in attendance, left to run and shout with their balloons in tow. Belinda's nephew Roy hovered over the grave with another little girl of about eight years of age. One of the balloons escaped, and instead of going up, it dragged near the ground just over the still open grave where Belinda's casket now sat. It even seemed to be tugged on, so that it bobbed up and down. Suddenly it popped.

Roy: (laughing) That's Belinda who did that!

Little Girl: (shaking her head and frowning) No it's not. She's dead!

Roy: No, she did that. I know she did.

Little Girl: (exasperated) But she's down there! (pointing)

Roy: I know, but she did it anyway. She playin' with us.

Other children gathered around, listening to this debate and peering down to see if Belinda had any more tricks to play. Andrena suddenly realized that Belinda didn't have her favorite backpack. She retrieved it and she dropped it on to the casket. Andrena joked through her tears: "You know, she's gonna need that pack. She's already opened it, to see what she's got in there. I can feel Belinda below me, pulling everything out of her purse, as I've seen her do a million times before." We continued to sing "Happy Birthday" as dirt was thrown on the casket, "I love you Belinda, I love you Belinda," Andrena repeated in a low moan over and over again. We all looked up to watch the balloons.

Some were snagged by the trees. Some just kept flying up, the exact color as the sky. Suddenly I could feel underneath me a whole child world, a children's playground as the balloons were floating up and out, well above the trees. Andrena commented quietly, "Belinda gave us a nice day for this. You know Belinda's looking down at us right now, smiling down at us."

Here is the emplotment of a funeral: the creation of a highly charged moment both orchestrated and improvised. It played upon and resisted the usual convention of space and time. In significant ways, it resisted the context as well as made use of it. This was a burial of an African American child in a very upscale white neighborhood. This potent emplotment transformed context in several ways. It remade a blank impersonal space, or even a mournful space, into an underworld child's playground, one where children (above the ground) could safely play with their dead. When Andrena gave us balloons and we let them go, the burial became not only a place to say good-bye but a moment of celebration, a letting-go in which Belinda was still very much alive. She even appeared apparitional at that moment of release when the balloons floated angelically up above us. At the same time, earthily below us, there was still that familiar mischievous and social girl who loved to rummage through her purses and enjoyed nothing better than playing tricks on her cousins.

Through this emplotment, Belinda's death emerged (even for me with all my religious skepticism) as a healing moment. Her burial did seem like a going-away party that celebrated a better phase of life, rather like sending a child off to college or even to kindergarten. While sad and very much an ending, Belinda's burial marked a beginning, too. I have been to many funerals, but I have never been to one in which I experienced a funeral as any kind of graduation, as a moment in which a hopeful future could still be promised. This experience was accomplished through story telling, through music, but especially through the visual and the kinesthetic, the dramatic shaping of time itself.

Though Andrena hoped for a cure, ultimately healing came to mean something very different. It marked, instead, another episode in a narrative where she herself was transformed from a distraught, even suicidal mother to someone who came to volunteer at the hospital where her daughter was treated, helping other parents whose children were critically ill. She became a guide through an unbearable journey.

Andrena did a number of things while Belinda was alive that helped her to construct "hope in the crossroads," so to speak. This crossroads marked three paths with their accompanying hopes: (1) hope her child would live, (2) hope she could find a reason to live even if her child died, and (3) hope that if her child died this could be a "good death" after a "good life," however brief. These paths are not only divergent but, in the case of the first two, are mutually contradictory. Furthermore, the cultivation of each of these paths feeds the task of narrative re-envisioning that Andrena set for herself soon after she confronted Belinda's diagnosis. There are two paths that Andrena feels morally impelled to avoid, and both of these "tempt" her when she begins the journey through suffering engendered by Belinda's illness. One is to "run away" rather than stay by Belinda's side through the illness. This is the unthinkable abandonment that she laments other family members did—most notably her husband. She would never physically leave her daughter. But for Andrena, abandonment is also seeing her daughter through despairing eyes, as though she were "already gone." The other path, she fears, will tempt her too much, that she will kill herself if her daughter does not live. Her determination to find some way to hope reveals her belief that hope is the only path that might lead her away from what she finds ethically untenable, her own self-destruction. However, hope that rests on the happy ending of cure is too flimsy. This will not do.

The task of narrative re-envisioning she undertakes propelled her to experimentally move *toward* death in order to embrace life. She "practiced" becoming intimate with death when she befriended Sashi and Drea. And she brought Belinda into this practice as well. In a telling exchange that painfully highlights this movement, Drea and Andrena once joked about how much of Drea's chicken Belinda ate on one of their visits. Andrena rejoiced at this rare moment when Belinda took pleasure in food, a greedy childish moment in the kitchen while another child lay in a coma in the next room. If this is to be a narrative of hope, hope itself must come to mean something different.

Her child's burial serves as a powerful instance of this reconfiguring of hope, a moment that allowed her to express and construct a hopeful vision of her child's past and future and of her own future as well. Belinda's funeral, in particular, was dramatically symbolic of Andrena's long work of re-envisioning. Andrena herself was transformed in this journey. Instead of thinking, as she did when Belinda was first diagnosed, that she would commit suicide if her daughter died, she came to a point where she would not only face this death but redouble her efforts to help other parents whose children were critically ill.

THE SPECTER OF MORAL TRAGEDY

Andrena struggled to cultivate virtues that would allow her to persevere and even thrive in the face of Belinda's death. But can she really go on, year after year, in a situation where she not only continues to mourn the death of her child but finds herself in difficult economic straits? The part-time job she had gotten, one she loved, chauffeuring a wealthy family's two boys around to their after-school activities, ended abruptly when they relocated back to Singapore. Time and again I would get a call from her, sometimes in the middle of the night, where she would simply break down. "It's too much Cheryl," she would cry. "What can I do?" I never knew what to say. I could see that she was staring straight into an abyss.

I return to her in the final chapter.

PART THREE

Moral Pluralism as Cultural Possibility

CHAPTER 7

Rival Moral Traditions and the Miracle Baby

In moral enquiry we are always concerned with the question: what type of enacted narrative would be the embodiment, in the actions and transactions of actual social life, of this particular theory? For until we have answered this question about a moral theory we do not know what that theory in fact amounts to; we do not as yet understand it adequately. And in our moral lives we are each engaged in enacting our own narrative, so revealing implicitly, and sometimes also explicitly, the not always coherent theoretical stance presupposed by that enactment. Hence differences between rival moral theories are always in key part differences in the corresponding narrative.

—(MacIntyre 1990:80)

A key agenda of critical theorists—problematizing the moral norms of everyday life—becomes, at times, an agenda of people everywhere when confronting moral dilemmas and tasks. In earlier chapters, I explored a range of cultural resources parents draw upon as they struggle to create good lives, or at least the best one possible, for their children. Up until this point, my primary analytic attention has been on how to conceptualize projects of moral becoming and attempts at transformation in a "thick" way that does justice to the complexity of these endeavors. I have said comparatively less, in a cultural or sociological vein, about the enduring features of the social spaces I have described.

This chapter and the following one represent a shift in emphasis. The social spaces themselves emerge more prominently as "main characters" and the narrativity I describe is less about narrative selves (though these are still in evidence) than about narrative practices. These two final ethnographic chapters showcase clashes of normative authorities and discourses, exploring how even the most valorized normative practices may be put under scrutiny and become, at least temporarily, unmoored. The chapters also consider the politics of care and moral becoming as they become intertwined with acts of overt resistance. In this one, I return to the clinic.

Every family in our study has stories to tell about how they have had to learn to challenge clinical care. The necessity of resistance came as a surprise to many parents, despite long familiarity with the crucial role of protest for the civil rights of black citizens. The surprise, for many of them, was that they would have to fight so assiduously for care and be so vigilant about it. None of them initially saw themselves as political activists, and most would still not adopt that label even though all have stories about how they have had to learn to practice what we on the research team came to call "just right non-compliance" (Mattingly 2010b). This involves such tactics as flouting rules where necessary to get clinical services, stealthily seeking second opinions when you believe a health problem needs more attention (as Dotty does with the pulmonologist), ignoring advice you think is bad but thanking the clinician for giving it, acting like you know less about your child's medical condition than you do so that you won't embarrass—and potentially alienate—a novice clinician, bringing small food gifts to hospital receptionists and nursing staff if you have argued too hard with them, taking care not to disagree with clinical staff so directly or vehemently that you risk jeopardizing your child's care, or worse yet, get a social worker "called on you," and a host of other strategies. Resisting or creatively improvising upon clinical moral norms was a necessary but often distasteful or wearisome job, often one parents shouldered reluctantly only because care of their children required it. As we saw with Dotty and also intimated by Tanya in the first chapter, it is a job that can come with high moral costs.

But sometimes moral critique and challenge are more direct and sustained. I explore some instances in this chapter and the following one. I look at how multiple and even rival moral schemes become resources for moral debate. Though I speak of these resources with attention to local moral communities specific to the African American families in our study, my claims are of a more general nature. As anthropologists have pointed out, social communities are unlikely to be morally homogenous; there will be multiple and even rival moral schemes and traditions in circulation. As noted in earlier chapters, studies of moral subjectivity in anthropology have revealed that people may well participate in practices that draw upon, work between, or even cultivate these rival moral schemes. Even within a single moral tradition there can be mechanisms for critique of the very institutions this tradition also supports. In other words, the practices that help reproduce a particular moral "regime of truth" will also contain within them resources with which they can be contested. This is the topic of chapter 8.

In this chapter I examine the co-presence of multiple moral traditions as these play out in a heated discussion about how to treat a critically ill infant. The baby's parents and clinicians enter into a sustained and often bitter battle about her care. One authoritative cultural space (the church and its religious practices) is pitched against another authoritative space (the clinic and its biomedical practices). These different traditions, as they are mobilized here, suggest an ontologically consequential divide. The terms of disagreement rest upon such profoundly different assumptions that a kind of moral incommensurability or, at the least a deep mutual misunderstanding, characterizes it, making it very difficult for the quarreling parties to recognize the terms of their difference.

Put starkly, their quarrel does not concern the same baby. For the parents, she is a living miracle. For the clinicians, or most of them, she is an unnatural artifact, a kind of machine hybrid that only *appears* to be a living infant. This ontological murkiness creates not only a moral impasse but also new moral possibilities as clinicians and parents debate her fate. We have become accustomed in anthropology and philosophy to contemplating the status of various kinds of machine–human assemblages. We often imagine a (posthuman) future populated by more and more cyborgic creatures who have transferred themselves from science fiction to science labs. Already these entities can be found in many places, including neonatal intensive care units. There is much public fascination and debate about them. But my purpose here is not to take up the moral issues surrounding this debate in a general (third person) way or to think in posthuman terms about what the invention of new human–machine relationships implies about the category of the ethical subject. Rather, I ask some very first person questions, especially from the parents' perspective: How is this baby a living miracle for them? What are her agentive and even specifically moral powers—how does she act on her parents in a moral way? How do these powers give her an "I" and bestow upon her a human status that the parents find irrefutable despite the clinician's competing claims?

These questions are culturally shaped. The perspective of the clinicians instantiates a particular set of theories, embedded in the culture of biomedicine, not only about illness, healing, and the body but also about what it means to be human. The parents' perspective manifests a rival theoretical position about all these matters that is culturally grounded especially in their religion. MacIntyre suggests that in the matter of moral debates between "fundamentally opposed standpoints" the outcome will inevitably be inconclusive, because there are a priori differences in cultural perspective that preclude the possibility of, for example, collecting sufficient empirical evidence to support one position and refute the alternative. "Each warring position characteristically appears irrefutable to its own adherents; indeed in its own terms and by its own standards of argument it is in practice irrefutable. But each warring position equally seems to its opponents to be insufficiently warranted by rational argument" (1990:7). As we shall see in this case, this inability to provide persuasive evidence to the opposing party does not prevent each side from amassing such evidence and presenting it to their opponents.

MacIntyre also remarks that "difference between rival moral theories are always in key part differences in the corresponding narrative" (1990:80), and this will certainly be evident in what follows. I consider how this very basic category, the "human," is challenged and defended through the use of implicit metaphors and enacted narratives that are embodied in actions, authoritative discourses, and the orchestration of physical space. I pay special attention to the narrative nature of the debate. Contestations between culturally normative discourses need not play themselves out as explicit arguments among competing points of view, of course. When we talk about moral theories as they operate in everyday life, we cannot refer only to propositional or verbally formulated statements of belief. Rather, it is necessary to look to the aesthetic, connotative, embodied manner in which theories are revealed. To explore the authority of both clinical and religious discourses, I examine the core cultural narratives and metaphors that are put into play, reimagined, and refigured in a series of charged interactions over the best good for this baby.

Attention to the poetics of normative social discourse and practice highlights its deeply imaginative character. When I opened this book with an experimental soccer field, I might have seemed to presume a prior social and physical space we could think of as "literal" or "real" or "just plain" soccer. But this misses something essential, because these too are imagined spaces. By this, I simply mean that even in their most routine incarnations and ritualized, predicable, and "literal" moments, social spaces and practices invoke and depend upon powerful cultural imaginaries; they are always already "figured worlds" (Holland et al. 1998). Moral experiments are not challenges to something literal so much as challenges to cultural imagination.

A NEONATAL INTENSIVE CARE UNIT

Andrew and Darlene's daughter, Arlene, was born with severe spina bifida and was immediately admitted into the neonatal intensive care unit (NICU). She was not expected to live long. She was kept alive only with sophisticated medical technology that sustained such essential life processes as her breathing, the circulation of blood, eating, and the like. At the family's insistence, she underwent close to thirty surgeries in the twenty-two months of her life in order to keep her alive. Some of these were highly experimental. She was never medically stable. There were a number of times when her heart stopped and clinicians had to revive her. These parents, who were deeply religious, found themselves in a difficult and ongoing confrontation with the clinicians caring for their child. From the parents' perspective, however, the clinicians were not merely performing clinical experiments but moral ones. For them, the NICU emerged as a moral laboratory in which their own religious faith was tested. It also became a kind of church in which they could practice and profess their faith to the skeptical clinicians. I have already introduced them in the previous chapter as Darlene, in particular, finds herself the target of Drea's angry words.

Although it is not infrequent for clinicians and families to find themselves in opposition about clinical care for their children, seldom in our study did we see a struggle so pitched and so prolonged as it was for this family. The most basic conflict between Andrew and Darlene and the clinicians was that the hospital staff was trying to get them to agree to a Do Not Resuscitate (DNR) decision the next time Arlene went into a medical crisis. They vehemently refused. For nearly two years, the parents and clinicians were locked in a heated battle over this DNR order. Several times during the twenty-two-month period that the child lived the clinicians warned the parents that she would die any minute, although this prognosis did not prove to be true on several of these occasions.

Despite the fact that her parents were sometimes told outright or in metaphorical terms that their infant was brain-dead ("Your child is just a vegetable"), this was not, legally speaking, quite the situation. Dr. Jewett, a senior physician on staff at the hospital, spoke about the complexities of this case. He made it clear that the hospital would very likely have taken legal action against the parents' wishes if it were legally warranted. "Now I guess my view is, if a child were brain-dead by the traditional accepted methodologies . . . if a family then refused to turn off the machines I guess my feeling is that we would leave a judge to do it. To get a court order to that effect." It was precisely the fact that Arlene did not meet the legal guideline for brain death, even though every system in her body was failing and she required extensive medical intervention to keep her alive, which created such a difficult situation for everyone concerned. Jewett is in agreement with the vast majority of clinical staff about the reasonableness of a DNR decision from a medical perspective: "Certainly a decision for a Do Not Resuscitate order would have been perfectly reasonable for the family to have accepted," but, he goes on to say, "it's the family's decision and their right to decide."

BIOMEDICINE'S METAPHORICAL IMAGINARY

Theorists like Lakoff and Johnson (1980) who have proposed that metaphor offers us an indispensable element of all our thinking are especially useful in exploring the pervasiveness and the tacit manner in which certain canonical metaphors have infiltrated routine medical care. In my own work in clinical settings, three primary metaphors have stood out: (1) healing as sleuthing; (2) healing as battling disease; and (3) healing as mechanical repair. In each of these, the body is represented metaphorically. It is variously a battleground, a crime scene, or a broken machine. All these metaphors are routinely employed in clinical encounters, often together (Mattingly 2010b). Root clinical metaphors like these are crucial and deeply embedded in the physical and social gestures of the clinic world. Each of these metaphors provides a core image around which particular clinical plots can be created—they are enacted and extended in the work of clinical care. That is, they provide the central image around which narratives are created. They also fuel definitive moral understandings of the good.

Anthropologists have provided critical commentary on the way that the "medicalization" of babies not only speaks to the culture of biomedicine but to "state discourses about what practices are considered 'respectable' versus 'pathological' for its citizens" (Craven 2005:194).

Although Dr. Jewett says that it is up to the family to decide—that is, it is their right (as citizens)—it will become increasingly clear that the clinical staff not only opposes the parents' decision but pathologizes them and questions this right. As Craven remarks, "Biomedical metaphors and beliefs about health that incorporate core American values, such as the authority of technological progress and mechanistic models of the body and its repair ... allow medical officials to assume an authoritative role regarding health care practices within the legislative arena" (2005:194–95).[1] Biomedicine's metaphors not only create links to legislative practices but also have the power to create "bad mothers" and "bad fathers." This has been of special consequence to African Americans, particularly the poor, who have been, for a number of historical reasons, singled out as *morally* lacking.[2]

In this chapter, I also look at how these parents challenge biomedical authority, especially one of its most valued and tacit metaphors—the body as machine.[3] As a machine, the body is potentially "fixable." This machine metaphor is not at all abstract, some mere scholarly conceit. It belongs to medical common sense, and more broadly, it is an implicit part of a cultural narrative of illness and healing. In canonical terms, the clinician (the surgeon as prototype here) operates as a kind of super-technician, a super-mechanic. "The institutional structure of health care, with its array of specialists, helps to keep a narrow focus on fixing certain body parts or improving their particular functions."[4]

The machine-body metaphor is invoked by clinicians and contested by these parents, who reimagine this trope within a spiritual discourse that offers competing authoritative metaphors and narratives. I look at how it is taken up, problematized, and even "poached" (to borrow de Certeau's [1984] felicitous term) by them. Although the machine metaphor operates virtually unnoticed in many clinical encounters, through the battle over both the DNR order and the family's insistence on doing everything medically necessary to keep their daughter alive, its troublesome metaphorical qualities as deployed in medical care become increasingly apparent.

This authoritative clinical metaphor, as Beardsley (1962, 1967) points out with regard to poetry, depends upon logical absurdity. Logical absurdities send us off in search of ways to save the sense of the sentence by foregrounding attributes of the one (machines) that are somehow similar to the other (humans). This might all sound very cognitive, but Ricoeur has another, and I think (again for my purposes) more apt way of describing what we are doing. These logical absurdities point us to different worlds, different imaginative spaces. If we follow Beardsley in speaking of metaphor as a logical absurdity—the body is not (logically speaking) literally a machine—then we begin to see, in its explicit employment, how both its limits and its absurdity are brought into sharp relief. Notably, this is not the kind of poetic absurdity that literary theorists find so promising, the way that it may afford semantic innovation, "producing a new semantic pertinence by means of an impertinent attribution," as Ricoeur puts it (1984:ix). He goes on to state, "The metaphor is alive as long as we can perceive, through the new semantic pertinence—and so to speak in its denseness—the resistance of the words in their ordinary use and therefore their incompatibility at the level of a literal interpretation of the sentence" (1984:ix).

A CONTESTED METAPHOR

In the following exchange, the machine-body indeed comes alive, resurrected from its usual tacit status, but what is revealed is not so much its imaginative possibilities as its dangers. One of Arlene's nurses is trying—yet again—to get the family to agree to a DNR decision. Although every part of the infant's body has been systematically failing, the nurse focuses upon problems with her heart to make her case. She explains to them that "the heart is not pumping correctly" and that it is getting increasingly difficult to keep the "lines" from her heart (her veins and arteries) open. Andrew resists the implications of her explanations, mentioning that he has heard that the doctors can "put a main line in" to help alleviate this problem. The nurse then resorts to an explicit and extended treatment of the machine-body metaphor: Arlene's body is an "old car," an old car with a bad engine. It is like but unlike a car the nurse owns, a beloved 1987 Toyota Tercel. They are both alike, presumably, in being machines that require a great deal of maintenance and working engines (or hearts); all the lines must work, must be in good repair, for them to go.

Her analogical reasoning seems to indicate that if her old car needed a new engine, it—like Arlene—would not be able to keep going. But, then she turns the analogy another direction. As it happens, her car and Arlene are unlike because if her Tercel needed a new engine, they could "plop" one in and it would still go because "the body in this car is still good." Arlene is a different matter, a more seriously malfunctioning machine. They can't drop another heart in because "her body is slowly giving out on us."

Nurse: Let me put it this way okay? I hate to use this analogy. But would you just bear with me a minute? I have a great car. I love it. It's an '87 Toyota Tercel. We've got over two hundred thousand miles [on it]. This car's got a motor and a heart that goes goes goes goes. I mean I adore this car. But I've got to make sure that everything works, and the lines, all the lines all the, [*Andrew:* Right] you know like everything in it. If something goes wrong in that car, I'm at the point—you know if it was still in good shape—but if I have to go and replace the engine and go plop another engine in it (she pauses) well, it'll go, because the body is still good. The body in this car is still good. Her body is slowly giving out on us. It's slowly giving up on us. And we can't drop another heart in.

Andrew: Yeah, well, well, that time haven't came yet.

The "logical absurdity" here is not about the extent to which Arlene is like an old car with a bad engine or an old car, like the Toyota in question, that could keep on running even with an engine/heart transplant. Rather, it is the machine metaphor altogether that is exposed (at least to the researchers) as absurd in the extreme. Is the love of these parents for their child the same as the nurse's love for her old car? Is the effort to keep her car maintained equivalent to the vigilance and even desperation they show at every turn to keep their child alive? Will they miss their daughter when she quits "running" or if they agree to "pull the plug" just the same as this nurse will miss her car when it finally dies?

The exchange that immediately follows Andrew's flat assertion that he is not persuaded by her "old car" metaphor is especially interesting. It exposes the internal battle that has been going on among the clinical staff; many strongly feel that the clinicians should not be doing all these operations and other "heroic measures" on this critically ill infant. In the following passage, the nurse reveals her stance on the matter, stating that the doctors "like to fight the mechanics." In other words, they are willing to fight or defy the natural mechanics of the body, making repair after repair quite beyond what one ought to do for a body-machine that is simply, inevitably giving out.

Nurse: No. We're pushing it. We're pushing it. We're pushing this real hard. And it's our procedure, we can't fight. (She pauses.) See, doctors like to fight the mechanics. 'Cause they read and they study, they know technology and everything. But what they will not acknowledge. (She pauses here, as though worried about how baldly she can put things.) Because this is (pausing again) . . . We're, we're going *beyond* what we usually do. (She smiles.)

Andrew: Well. (He shrugs and says nothing.)

What the nurse seems to be suggesting—and what is made explicit by many of the staff—is that the doctors have created an "artificial baby." It is not "natural" to extend her life in this way. Although the machine-body metaphor is regularly employed by clinicians to suggest that through various kinds of medical procedures—including the use of machines and all manner of advanced technology—the body's mechanical capabilities can be augmented, there is a limit to this. At some point, this limit will be reached and the child will inevitably die. A number of clinicians emphasized this perspective, arguing that what the staff were doing in their surgeries and through the use of external machines, had become unnatural. For example, a supervising physician who was very involved with the family expressed her anxieties about her own clinical interventions and what the hospital was doing as a whole in these terms:

> I've literally never met such a medically dependent child, and this is at this hospital [which treats highly involved medical cases] . . . Her airways cannot even stay open. She has stents to keep the airways open. That is not—to me, that is just, like, so artificial—so unnatural. Cannot breathe on her own. I mean, you know, it's just so many things that to me, it's just been a sign, and I feel this is so artificial and [sigh], talking with one of the residents—actually a couple of the residents who have seen what she has gone through all these times, you know, it's really—you know, it's numerous blood tests, all sorts of procedures, all sorts of operations . . . being suctioned, all this. . . . [She sighs again and shakes her head.]

To give another illustration of the limits of the machine-body metaphor from a clinical perspective, in the following exchange, a surgeon, Dr. Sanderson, draws upon the imagery of body as broken machine to try to impress upon Andrew and Darlene that their baby should be taken off life support. One can hear almost desperation in Dr. Sanderson's relentless cataloguing of body breakdowns "from head to toe" and how deeply the machine imagery is embedded in the clinical imaginary. He seems to be trying to convey to the parents that their daughter has become too much of a machine, that the failure of her internal machinery in so many critical functions and her reliance on these external machines means she is, in effect, dead. (A more extended version of this conversation is found in Mattingly 2010b:71–72.) He begins in the following way.

> I want to start by describing her conditions from head to toe. I have spent quite a bit of time with her and have seen her progress. I want to start with her lungs. She no longer breathes by herself. Several times during the day, we have to bag her for long periods of time just to bring her back from death.

Sometimes the ventilator is not enough because her body is making so many secretions they are blocking the lungs and airways. Her stents which have been replaced several times are collapsing down and might be clogging her lungs. . . . In order to just get rid of the secretions, we have to detach her from the machine, which makes her desaturate. Her vent settings are almost at their maximum and for someone her size, so much pressure damages the lungs more and more. Her lungs are getting worse and worse and it's harder and harder to keep her alive. . . . Another thing is her heart. Her heart is beating slower and slower. Because of her heart disease, it needs to work harder to pump blood through her body. When the lungs are bad, it's harder and harder on her heart. We could try to fix the heart, but she wouldn't survive the surgery. So to fix her heart is not an option. You have that going downhill too.

He continues to report her various failing systems and why there is no good medical solution for them. The conversation between Andrew and Dr. Sanderson that follows the doctor's lengthy explanation reveals moral pluralism at work.

> *Dr. Sanderson:* What I ask myself every time I walk into her room is, "Am I doing the best thing for this child?" That's the question I ask myself.
>
> *Andrew:* Yes. Yes. We don't want to take her off the machines. When she goes, she's going to go on her own. That's how I believe. That's how she'll fight it out.
>
> *Dr. Sanderson:* As long as you know that it's not her, but the machines that are keeping her alive.
>
> *Andrew:* The only thing stopping her from dying is the machines and medicine. We understand that.

Andrew's response confounds the clinicians. Although he appears to agree with the doctor about the facts of the matter, "the only thing stopping her from dying is the machines and the medicine," he does not come to the same moral conclusion about the best good for his child.

In turning to the parents' perspective as a contrast to the way the clinicians see the child, I suggest that their moral reasoning differs so radically because it is embedded within a different, even incommensurable, narrative. If, as Ricoeur contends, metaphors are ostensive, if they point to a world beyond them, then the worlds to which this same metaphor points is not only distinctive but in many respects antithetical. I have already said something about the narrative horizon to which their machine-body refers from a canonical clinical perspective. One of its most important features, vividly shown in this situation, concerns the limits of this horizon. There comes a place at which mechanical interventions change the status of the body from natural to artificial, the clinicians are saying. A defective body-machine can only be rebuilt so far and then it ceases to be a body; it is humanly dead and literally becomes just a machine.

What seems so unnatural to clinicians is, by contrast, evidence to Andrew and Darlene that their daughter is a "miracle baby." God has found a way, even through the hands of clinicians who are unbelievers, to keep their child alive. God has resurrected her when clinicians believed her to be dead. When they consider their daughter's machine-body and the many machines used to augment it, they consider this as a manifestation of the creativity of God. God has created humans who have created machines, including those that keep their child alive. The practice of medicine and its machinery constitutes just a short story in a cosmological narrative. From their perspective, the clinicians simply misunderstand their own role in human history. They seem to believe that they (or these parents) should be in charge of life and death. But this is not a human matter. It is about hoping, struggling to hope, doing everything possible to sustain life while at the same time recognizing that life and death are not fully under human control. For them, the practice of healing invokes a plot that brings in an array of cosmological actors. This narrative not only encompasses the personal, the interpersonal, or the clinical—it is on a scale such that all of human history and its creations make up one small episode in a much vaster epic.

In reflecting on the metaphors and narrative plots mobilized in this conflict, one might be tempted to contrast the parents' religious metaphors and the cosmological narrative with a picture of biomedicine that traffics in scientifically grounded facts and statistically calculated risks. It might seem that religious reasoning relies in a special way upon metaphors and narratives, that it is *figural* in a way that science (and its application in biomedicine) is not. However, I suggest that both the discourse of biomedicine and alternative lay discourses (religion, in this case) are suffused with morally consequential metaphors.

Biomedical practices and the logic of their reasoning are equally dependent upon figural infrastructures, upon underlying metaphors and narratives. *Because* practical sciences like medicine appear to deal in facts, in what turns out to be (probabilistically) true, the metaphorical and symbolic are less readily apparent. And when, in a situation like the one I've described, the metaphorical understanding of the body as machine actually surfaces *as* a metaphor, it may seem absurd, even scandalous. It can't be that a child, however broken, is the same as a Toyota Tercel, after all. It might be tempting to blame an inept nurse for this misstep in communication (not to speak of empathy), but this is missing the point. Instead of singling out a particular practitioner, one might ask, what culturally, within the practice of biomedicine, makes this analogy work? Why is it so morally persuasive?[5] Such questions have been subtly addressed by scholars from a range of disciplines (including science and technology studies, medical anthropology and medical humanities). I won't try to say much more about them here. Rather, I turn to the moral framework that Andrew and Darlene embrace. How does their moral reasoning, so baffling to the clinicians, reflect a ground project of care and a moral experiment in their own projects of becoming?

THE SPIRITUAL IMAGINARY AND
THE CULTIVATION OF WISDOM

For Darlene and Andrew, their child is part of a story of transformation that encompasses both their particular personal and family history narratives and a cosmological scene. They spoke repeatedly about how Arlene had brought "sobriety" to them and a recommitment to religious practices. Although they saw biomedicine and biotechnology as essential for their child's care, they also believed medical practices should be combined with spiritual ones. Their perspective was that although doctors were skilled at some things, they as parents could also cultivate practices that could improve their daughter's chances. Thus, they did not see their task as merely receiving the clinicians' diagnoses about the child's state. Rather, through prayerful dwelling upon stories from "God's book," and through lengthy prayer, they could help to bring God's power onto the scene. This might even result in miraculous curing. In this way, they too, could actively assist in the production of healing, albeit through a very different avenue. When at one point the doctors told them that their child was a "vegetable," Andrew responded by intensifying his prayer practices, even recruiting his children to help. He once told us, "I can see that we serve only one God, and He's a powerful God. And Sunday, me and the boys we went to church, we sat in that church from eleven to seven praying, you know."

If there is a moral incommensurability between Andrew's and Darlene's religious narrative of their miracle baby and the clinical narrative of an artificial machine baby, this does not illustrate some form of exotic cultural relativism, however. Rather, their conflict reflects a moral pluralism that runs so deep in American society that it can create fundamental ontological schisms, obstructing any easy translation from one vocabulary to another. Andrew and Darlene's response, the narrative to which they are committed, is at once a personal story and a very American one. Americans as a whole are famously religious, with close to 95 percent of them professing belief in some kind of divine power.[6] While obviously many religious Americans would not make the moral choices that Andrew and Darlene do, or see their child in the same way (Drea, for example, sees things differently), these parents draw upon imagery and beliefs that are culturally inflected.

Their Christian tradition provides cultural resources that they draw upon, although it certainly does not predetermine the moral choices that they make. They are not simply *following* a religion, in other words. It is more accurate to say that their Christianity affords them the cultural possibility to see their infant as a miracle baby. It guides them, pedagogically, in practices intended to strengthen their spiritual faith and their wisdom to perceive and judge what is best for their child. Their judgments are deeply intertwined with their own individual and familial life journeys. For them, Arlene has a special role to play, especially for Andrew, because she, unlike any of their other children, has been powerful enough to bring him back to God. Or, as they would see it, God has been able to speak to Andrew and Darlene through the gift of this terribly ill baby.

What, then, are some of the cultural resources their Christianity provides? For one, it brings them back into a church community that offers them strong support.[7] Extended families and the church arguably constitute the two most dominant, well-established, and influential social institutions in many African American communities.[8] The church has been especially important for poor African Americans from the rural South, places like the small town in Louisiana where Andrew was born and raised.[9] Andrew and Darlene practice and experience their spirituality in an intensely emotional and individual way, as connected to the personal relationship they cultivate with Jesus, especially through the practice of prayer. This, too, has cultural roots, which go beyond the African American experience, speaking to a broadly shared American evangelical tradition (Luhrmann 2012). Jesus, in particular, plays a dominant role as a deity with whom one can form a personal relationship.[10] The relational component of black religious experience and expression encompasses God, one's community, and one's ancestors as well.[11] The Bible is not simply read literally so much as read in relationship to one's own personal experiences, including direct revelations from God. Prayer is essential for cultivating one's spirituality. And for many African Americans, an active practice of prayer is necessary to learn other virtues, including humility and faith that enable one to turn matters over to God (Grant 1989). For Andrew and Darlene, as for many other families in our study, the idea of "turning it over to the Lord" is an essential aspect of facing serious illness.[12] The practice of prayer is paramount in caring for one's health or the health of loved ones; many devout Christians believe that it can have direct practical consequences on one's health.[13]

Abrums (2000), who writes with wonderful subtlety about the intersection of race, religion and health, describes how the body was conceived among the African Americans she studied at a storefront church. Her depiction is so congruent with Andrew's and Darlene's perspective that I follow her closely here. Like the people Abrums studied, Andrew and Darlene distinguished intelligence gained from experience and from the cultivation of proper emotions (what Aristotle would call wisdom) from intellectual book learning. For Abrums's informants, too, it is the former that was especially prized and it involved a training of the heart. "There were many traditional black sayings that addressed this same issue. A visiting preacher said, 'up here will fool you (pointing to his head), in here will school you' (pointing to his heart)" (2000:98). This kind of distinction gives a particular centrality to the body and to healing. "One had to understand that Jesus was in charge of the body. . . . The 'intelligent' person recognized the most essential meaning of the body, that it was a beautiful gift from God, given so that one could know God. The intelligent person also held another truth, that only God had power over the body" (2000:98).

bell hooks, using very similar language, recounts the words her grandmother told her before she set off for Stanford from her poor home in Kentucky:

> Indeed one crucial value that I had learned from Baba, my grandmother, and other family members was not to believe that "schooling made you smart." One could have degrees and still not be intelligent or honest. I had been taught in a culture of poverty to be intelligent, honest, to work hard, and always to be a person of my word. I have been taught to stand up for what I believed was right, to be brave and courageous. . . . These lessons were the foundation that made it possible for me to succeed. . . . They were taught to me by the poor, the disenfranchised, the underclass. (1994:167)

Book learning, by itself, is insufficient for the cultivation of true intelligence or wisdom because it can be divorced from both practical action and from training the heart. The contrast with biomedicine's view of knowledge is striking. Within the clinical moral imaginary, knowledge is separated from personal practice or moral virtue so profoundly that it makes perfect sense for an expert medical practitioner to have the knowledge to treat her patients even if she herself lives an unhealthy life.

Similarities between virtue ethics (especially a first person kind) and this religious understanding of knowledge and moral life are readily apparent here. The separation between knowledge and practice that characterizes modern understandings of expertise was not possible in Aristotle's age, for example. Medicine, like all aspects of everyday life, was associated with notions of virtue. There is a shared focus in this religious perspective and ancient ethics on cultivating virtues as integral to moral decisions and actions, an understanding of moral becoming as part of a journey, an emphasis on the essential role of personal experience in cultivating virtues, and the presence of "technologies" (to use Foucault's language) to be learned and regularly practiced in order to enable this process (e.g., in the religious case, prayer, reading the Bible, attending church). There is also a shared belief that humans are not "self-sufficing" but part of an order that also includes higher and more powerful beings to whom humans are expected to give respect and reverence, a view that ethical and even other kinds of knowledge are dependent upon the knower, the one who practices and cultivates virtues.

Charles Taylor notes the enormous difference between antiquity's virtue ethics and modern medicine. Taylor remarks:

> We are in a different universe from that of, say, Aristotelian ethics, where a concept like 'phronesis' doesn't allow us to separate a knowledge component from the practice of virtue. This becomes possible with modern science, construed as knowledge of an objectified domain, as with our contemporary Western medicine. Even more striking, this recourse to objectified knowledge begins in modern culture to take over ethics (Taylor 2007:501).

But this does not mean that this ancient ethics is completely foreign to contemporary life. If there are certain resonances between the religious perspective that Darlene and Andrew rely upon and the virtue ethics of antiquity, this is not by sheer chance. Mahmood (2005) connects the practices and beliefs of contemporary religious Islamic women to virtue ethics by making the historical case that Aristotelian thought was imported into Islam hundreds of years ago. One could argue with equal plausibility that Christian practices bear vestiges of an Aristotelian outlook that they absorbed through the influence especially of Augustine and Aquinas.[14] Obviously the worlds of the ancient Greeks and present-day African American Christians are extremely different.

And yet, we see a number of shared assumptions, especially when we contrast these virtue ethics traditions with moral perspectives associated with the practices of science, technology, medicine, and modernity's ethics. Taylor's portrait of the contrast helps explain why Andrew and Darlene and the clinicians have such difficulty finding a shared moral vocabulary from which to persuasively make their cases.

THE TRANSFORMATIVE JOURNEY OF ANDREW AND DARLENE

Because of their strong religious beliefs, it might appear that this family did not suffer the same struggle for hope that Dotty, Sasha, Andrena, or other families experienced. But this is not at all the case. Andrew and Darlene often talked about how difficult it was to have the strength to care for their daughter and to suffer with her without themselves giving up. Andrew spoke of this once, his prose a kind of prayer, having just arrived at the hospital to see Arlene. Although he tells us that both his daughter and the clinician need him and his prayers, he finds this task almost unbearable:

> "Lord, please help me. Help me Jesus. They [the clinicians] need you." You know, but it's, it's just so, it's just so much. [He sighs as he recalls how difficult it was to face his baby day after day.] I'm glad the good Lord has strengthened us and made us able. You know, because He, the good Lord He, He ain't going to give us ones that we can't help. He knows He can't give the ones we can't help. And that's the way He wrote it down for me, and for my wife to happen.

Andrew remembers how far he and his wife have come on their own spiritual journey, a journey they needed to take to be able to care for such a critically ill child. Their passage has been made only through the help of Jesus. As Andrew sometimes puts it, "We came from a long way." Once he and his wife had been heavy drinkers and drug users, but they had "turned to Christ." Andrew, especially, spoke eloquently about how this child "brought him to Jesus" and helped him overcome a long history of drug use. Instead of going to AA (Alcoholics Anonymous) meetings, he says, they used spiritual practices to overcome their addictions. Jesus "lightened me up," Andrew stated. Having been lightened, he and his wife could take on the burden of a daughter who, for two years, hovered near death until she was finally "healed" in heaven.

To cultivate an attitude of hope, Andrew and Darlene steeped themselves in biblical stories, prayerfully meditating upon religious figures who had also faced hard times or even, like Jesus, been required by God to embrace death itself. Dwelling upon stories of biblical characters who had also suffered and been redeemed offered an avenue for cultivating a certain kind of vulnerability, an ability to "wait and float and be actively passive," as Nussbaum puts it. These stories also served as lessons that Andrew and Darlene drew upon to deepen their compassion for their sick child, to stand by their daughter no matter what the cost.

But stories entered into their lives and moral practices in a more complex way. Just as Andrew and Darlene were compelled to undergo their own narrative re-envisioning in order to care for their child—turning away from drugs and giving their hearts to Jesus—so they felt that clinicians (especially doctors) had an analogous transformative journey ahead of them. It was not drugs that they saw as a moral impediment to the clinicians but hubris, a false pride in their own power. The family's strongly held view was that doctors also needed to have a change of character, a change of heart.

Andrew and Darlene spent a great deal of time not only telling clinicians stories that they hoped would work upon their hearts but also trying to enact a story of religious humility and belief in God that would engender a moral transformation among clinicians. A primary proof of such transformation, from their perspective, would be that clinicians would also recognize that they were "not God" and it was not up to them to make decisions over their daughter's life or death. They too should be willing to wait, vulnerably, thinking and acting "positive" (that is, doing everything they medically could for the child) but also recognizing that whether this little girl lived or not was in God's hands.

As we know, their spiritual perspective put them at odds with most (although not all) of the clinicians who treated Arlene, including religiously inclined staff. The parents were well aware of this and thus they saw their task in caring for their child as a task of counterpersuasion, or at least of religious witnessing. Strong critiques of Western medicine are voiced in some of their stories, both in its neglect of the spiritual and because without a spiritual perspective, clinicians lose a broader framework from which to understand illness and the nature and possibilities of healing. Christian beliefs and, specifically, beliefs in the power of God, are called upon to contest the grim prognoses of clinicians. God, they will often say, not the doctor, is ultimately in charge of life and death.

As evidence of the validity of such a stance, these parents cited past experiences when their own faith has proved them a better predictor of their children's fate than the scientific (and nonspiritual) knowledge they attributed to the doctors. Andrew told the following story not as a single event but as a recurrent one:

> The doctors would say, "Bring the whole family up here. She's going to die. This is her last day." You know, we fed off of that. . . . And [then] something told us . . . that baby ain't going nowhere. It's amazing, you know? You listen to them doctors, and then you get scared.

Darlene remembered a particular crisis with her critically ill little girl when she was three months old:

> They [the doctors] gave my daughter four days. It was January 1st. It was on a Thursday. They told me before that Monday, my daughter would die. They called the funeral home. The funeral home called the hospital to make arrangements—everything. They told me to cut off my daughter's hair. And I kept telling them, "No, no. She's not going. I don't feel like she's going." I kept praying for the grace of God to help me, strengthen me because I wasn't ready. [And now] . . . she's eighteen months old.

Andrew recalled a later moment when Arlene was declared "gone" by the clinicians but was later resuscitated. He told this story:

> I told the doctor when the doctor told me that my child was gone, I said, "Doctor, who are you? Who are you? You aren't even nobody. God put you here to do your work, but once God say your time is up, your time is up." But me and myself, as being a dad—what I think all parents should do is get your kids christened. Take them to church. Give them back to God.

Because their doctors did not incorporate a spiritual position into their professional framework, Andrew and Darlene had an added responsibility to bring this perspective into the clinic. Notably, they did not view biomedicine as *alternative* to, or in *contest* with, spiritual practices. Both were essential for physical healing. Given the nonspiritual orientation of their daughter's clinical services, the parents were more than willing to share the burden of effort. They would do the praying, reading of the Great Book, and other spiritual practices, helping to bring God's power to bear on the fate of their child in a miraculous way, and the doctors could call on their clinical books and their technology to do their part. They strongly believed that if the doctors would only come around to their perspective, then they would realize that they should do all within their "naturalistic" power to keep their daughter alive although all—doctors, parents, baby—awaited God's plan. God might either heal their child miraculously and allow her to physically get well, or "heal her in heaven" when he deemed that it was "her time."

Their unrelenting efforts created great consternation in the clinical team. Since the clinicians could not dissuade the family of their DNR decision, they had lengthy team meetings and many internal arguments about what their response should be. One of the most fascinating aspects of this case were instances, sometimes witnessed by us on the research team, sometimes told and retold by parents, when the clinicians themselves expressed astonishment that this baby, who they thought had "died," was still alive after all. The parents saw this as agentive; their child was teaching the doctors about the wisdom and power of God through her own miraculous recoveries, even, apparently, rising from the dead. Such a recovery, of course, recalls the most astonishing healing stories of the Bible, such as the rising of Lazarus or of Christ himself.

These events generated further stories that parents told clinicians, researchers, and themselves, providing narrative reinforcement of their path. The following one, co-narrated by both parents, recounts one vivid moment when their faith helped them to "convert" some of the doctors. In the following passage, I offer some key segments of their story. It begins with a call from the hospital, a call from a clinical department (most likely social work) that helps families with funeral arrangements. Darlene, the primary narrator, began telling the story:

Darlene: [The hospital] had the lady that arranges for the burial and everything. She called us and told us we would only have to pay for the transportation and the headstone and all that. And I was like, "Well, she ain't dead." She said, "Well most babies they send me, they be dead already." And I was like, "Well no, my daughter's not dead." But they still had her call us and stuff. . . . They had pronounced my baby dead to this lady.

Andrew: Then that woman turned around and called us the same night. "Well where do you want to bury your daughter at?" I said, "My baby's not even dead. Why are you asking that?"

Most of the clinicians unsurprisingly reject this narrative and the part the parents asked them to play in it. Several of them accused the parents of being selfish and unethical. In the following excerpt from an interview, Darlene speaks angrily about this. She is especially incensed and injured that while she and her husband believe they are acting out of faith, out of an ethical position they have struggled to maintain through prayers and calling upon God, the clinicians accuse them of an ethical breach, of being selfish in trying to keep their daughter alive.

Darlene opens this part of their story in the voice of one of her daughter's doctors:

> That doctor told us, "You guys need to start accepting." "Stop praying and start . . ." And I said, "No, no, no." I said, "You never stop praying." "Huh?" he said, "You all need to start accepting." No, what did he say?

She pauses, trying to remember his exact words.

> "Stop hoping and start accepting, because she's dead. . . ." They told me that we were being selfish for not pulling the plug on my daughter. I said, "I'm not pulling nothing on my daughter. Nothing!" He said, "So what do you think about that baby just laying there being a vegetable. That's selfish. She's dead. Her brain is dead. You need to pull the plug and get it over with and start accepting it." And I said, "I don't need to start accepting nothing! You better get away from me!" I was so mad. You know, he hurt my feelings. I was like, you know, how can you tell me something like that? That's my daughter. I want to hold on to her for as long as I can. If God ain't killing her, ain't no way I'm pulling the plug.

Darlene and Andrew remember the clinical staff telling them that they could hold their daughter "while she goes" when they "pulled the plug." To this, Darlene narrates her retort: "I said, 'I can hold her every day now, you know, and breathe with this plug for her.' You know what I mean? 'No, I don't want to pull the plug.' [The doctor] said, 'Well, it's up to you guys. It's you all's decision.'"

At this point, the history they recount in various interviews takes a dramatic turn. For, after this medical crisis in which all these confrontations occurred, their daughter revived. Although for nearly all her young life, she could not breathe without the aid of a ventilator, she improved sufficiently such that she was able to do so. Darlene and Andrew recount how the doctors came back to them, apologizing and confessing that they had been wrong. They had presumed Arlene was dead (brain-dead), but her ability to breathe on her own showed she was not, that she had more brain activity than they had anticipated.

Darlene, recalling "the same doctor" who had told them they were being selfish and that they needed to let their child go, gave the following account:

> And then the same doctor came and said, "This is a miracle. I don't understand why. . . ." He said, "But you guys were right. You guys knew your baby, and I am so sorry." He said, "This is a miracle." He said, "This is going to go down in history." He said he had to go to his higher people to tell them that what he told us, so that they can make it clear in the book that they did

pronounce the baby dead. He said they were going to write that in the book, that she was dead, but he had to go back and tell them that she wasn't.

What is particularly intriguing is that two books are juxtaposed here—a spiritual one and a clinical one. The clinical one is explicitly mentioned—it is a book that records clinical events, a clinical history. The revival of their baby constitutes a kind of medical miracle, an event that "is going to go down in history." But this medical miracle recalls miracles of a spiritual sort, miracles in which God even raises the dead. Thus, "the [clinical] book" provides an echo of the Great Book of God. This implicit reference to the Bible takes on material presence because all the while their daughter was kept alive in the NICU through a network of complex machinery connected to many parts of her body, her parents left an open Bible next to her head. It was remarkable to see this infant so completely surrounded by a complex technological web of wires and tubes and beeping machines while the Bible was also nestled on her pillow next to her. In the story Darlene tells with her husband, it is the active presence of the two books together that kept their daughter alive, against all medical odds.

In a later part of the interview, Darlene returns to this moment and the doctor's response to the reawakening of their daughter:

> The doctor says he's never seen a case like that in his life. But it's not for him to question. It came from Jesus. We prayed. Everybody prayed. I prayed to God that I was strong enough that He wouldn't take my daughter. "Please don't take my daughter yet." You know? And He didn't. He made her better.

In subsequent interviews, this "doctor conversion" story is told and retold by the parents. Andrew tells us how he needs to keep educating the doctors, who are blinded by their own knowledge. "All of them went to college, and they was wrong this time." Andrew notes that this even shook their faith in their own wisdom. This experience with his daughter "had themselves doubting." When one doctor expresses surprise at his daughter's continuing to live, Andrew explains to him that he sends God in as well as the doctor to help his daughter. "And the doctor says, man, how this baby do this here?" Andrew responds to him, "Because I sent her in there with Somebody. I don't just send her in there with you; I send her in there with Somebody else, too."

In one of the most explicit renderings, Darlene tells us:

> That doctor said, "Well, she can't handle no more." I said, "What do you mean she can't handle no more? Our God is powerful." We had to go show

them. . . . All of them [the doctors] came back after she came back [was able to breathe on her own] and they apologized real nicely. They said, "You know, we thought that we knew our stuff. But we see now that it is Somebody higher than us. And your family showed us that."

This conversion narrative, so steeped in biblical images and plot structures, is quite different than stories the clinicians told us about these recoveries. They spoke in much more ambiguous language. But many expressed shock at the baby's recoveries, and at the resilience of this little girl who, though she did die, lived much longer than anticipated and seemed to pull through crisis after crisis, surgery after surgery, despite their predictions. Some even privately pulled the parents aside and told them they were praying for her at their own churches.

Although the physician conversion that Andrew and Darlene recount was not as apparent to us as researchers, a conversion of a different sort did occur. In experiencing the steadfast spiritual witnessing of these parents, their constant attendance at the hospital, the tenderness with which they held their daughter, many clinicians did have a change of heart. Some who had initially dismissed those parents as "uneducated" or even selfish came to respect them. In fact, it seemed that Andrew and Darlene gained more respect even among clinicians who vehemently disagreed with their decisions than other families who did not set out to "convert" clinical staff. This change of heart among some of the staff reinforced to Andrew and Darlene that they were becoming and should continue to become better spiritual people so that they would be strong enough to care for their child.

SUBVERTING METAPHORS: HOW METAPHORS ARE POACHED IN CREATING A MIRACLE BABY

We can see in the challenges mounted by Andrew and Darlene the political force of religious discourse.[15] The focus on virtue as *both* a moral and political necessity is vivid in black church traditions. The African American Christian Church has been immensely important in providing a space for critiquing American civil society and authority, offering resources for mobilizing the poorest of the poor to stand up against powerful legal and social institutions (West 2008). One's spiritual allegiance not only provides a way to combat the powerlessness that racism afflicts, but to addresses the issue of social class as well. Poverty itself need not preclude one from having a voice.[16] This is no small thing for Andrew and Darlene, who are "ghetto," as Darlene joked more than once. W. E. B. Du Bois linked political protest and the cultivation of virtue (especially dignity) in explicit and vivid prose early in the twentieth century. He posed the questions: "How shall Integrity face Oppression? . . . What shall Virtue do to meet Brute Force?" Du Bois is asking, What could virtue offer in the face of black political invisibility and namelessness, in the face of being a "problem" for America?[17] A dominant African American religious response has been a steeped in spiritual imagery, what West calls the "prophetic utterance" (1996:90).

I conclude this chapter by considering more explicitly how Andrew and Darlene exhibit prophetic utterance in their use of clinical metaphors. They learn to become politically adept at holding to their position, despite immense pressure. The machine-body and other metaphors are rhetorically both invoked and reimagined by them in their contestations. They don't merely "consume" these clinical metaphors but "poach" them. This consumption of biomedicine involves acts of imaginative appropriation in which Andrew and Darlene creatively remake and reinterpret the oral and written words of clinicians and incorporate them within their own narratives of miraculous recoveries, the power of faith, and the centrality of meditative prayer. The stories they tell and the narrative horizon to which their metaphors and stories point embeds clinical practice within God's practice.

To illustrate this creative appropriation, I offer an example from a different metaphor frequently employed by clinicians as they try to persuade parents to "give up" on their child and "let her go naturally." In this instance, one of the nurses tells them that their child is a "vegetable."[18] In response, Darlene retorts if her daughter is a vegetable, she will be her garden. The home health nurse, Florence (one of the very few clinicians who supports the parents in both their religious perspectives and their decision over the DNR issue) listens supportively.

> *Darlene:* Let me tell you, Shanna [her primary nurse] said, "Your daughter's going to be a vegetable." I said, "That's okay, we're going to be her garden."
>
> *Florence:* I know that's worked.
>
> *Darlene:* Everybody, her brothers and her sister, is going to water her with no problems. We tell her she's going home with us. We going to be her garden and they're going to be the sprinklers. And she will grow.

In the usual version of this metaphor the relevant semantic domain invoked is what separates animals from vegetables as life forms; like a vegetable, the child lacks a brain. Both are "dead" in regard to brains.

In the mother's retort, she "poaches" this metaphor and offers an opposing response by shifting the semantic selection and highlighting other qualities of vegetables. They live in gardens. They are cultivated. They are watered. They are not only alive; they even grow if they are cared for. The fact that Darlene recognizes this as a political move, an act of rhetorical resistance, is clear not only in her manner of telling but in the home health nurse's appreciative response. "I know that worked."

Similarly, the machine-body metaphor is also creatively commandeered. In one of our earliest meetings with this family, Darlene introduced her daughter (who was then in the NICU) by pointing carefully to all of the different syringes that were used on her, the various medicines lined up along the side table, explaining what each was used for. She took a great deal of time pointing out all the monitors that were connected, through a maze of wires going to and from Arlene's body, again explaining what each machine was doing. Finally she lifted the blanket from her daughter's feet, showing the crocheted booties that she was wearing. As she shows the medicines, the machines, the wires, the booties, she repeats, "And this is her; this is her, this is her." The poaching is evident here in the act of pointing itself and her insistence that all these are part of Arlene. One would not ordinarily, in introducing one's child, point to each body part—the arms, the head, the legs, et cetera—and state again and again, "And this is Johnny, this is Johnny, this is Johnny." Of course it would be understood that all of these belonged to Johnny, *were* Johnny. Darlene recognizes that she is gesturing to a way of seeing her baby as a machine-body that places these machines within the circumference of the daughter. She is altering the canonical gaze, retracing the contours of her child's body. The poetry of her response relies upon claiming the machine body in all its material sensuality. In her pointing, she extends her child's body to include all the surrounding technologies that provide her life. Just as the machinery within the body supports life (or does ordinarily)—lungs that breathe, hearts that pump—so these machines have become her lungs, her heart, her stomach, her mouth. The machines are "naturalized" in a miracle body that can include all the artifacts that God has helped the doctors create.

CHAPTER 8

Dueling Confessions

Revolution in the First Person

Expectation, hope, intention towards possibility that has still not become: this is not only a basic feature of human consciousness, but, concretely corrected and grasped, a basic determination within objective reality as a whole.

—(Bloch 1986:7)

The world is possibility if only you'll discover it.

—Ralph Ellison, *Invisible Man* (1952:121)

THE MURDER

Leroy was not the first child in our study to die, but his death was the most unexpected. I first found out about his murder through Olga Solomon, one of the researchers on the team who had been close with the whole family for several years. Leroy's mother Marcy had just phoned her and announced that Leroy had passed away that day in a local hospital. I was stunned. Violence was not an uncommon occurrence for some of the poorer families residing in rough neighborhoods. Certainly it had been part of this family's life. But this, the sudden death of a boy I had known since he was six years old, one of the few who had seemed to be thriving, I wasn't prepared for it. And neither was his family.

I originally introduced Leroy, grandson of Delores, in a physical therapy outpatient clinic (chapter 3). Although his problem gradually diminished, other medical problems arose. He had always been stocky, but in his early teens he gained a great deal of weight, developed diabetes, and was put on insulin to control it. During this time, Marcy was serving time in prison for dealing drugs, although she remained clean.

(Three members of the household, Marcy, Sasha, and Leroy's older brother Ralph, were sometimes involved in this business. It was a major source of family income.) Delores, now very ill with breast cancer, could not take him to his doctor's appointments. His diabetes, left untreated, grew worse. When Marcy was released from prison, she brought him back to the doctors and the two of them went on a diet together. (She too suffered from diabetes.) In a few months his illness was under control and he no longer needed medication.

Leroy's murder occurred just after Delores died. Even during the worst stages of her illness, she continued to act as the matriarch and moral compass upon whom everyone relied. The last two years of her life she spent in a wheelchair, but she would not talk about her cancer. When we on the research team asked how she was feeling, she invariably smiled and said, "Oh, I'm fine. Doing okay," though it was clear she was very sick. The family was devastated by her death. The dynamics of the household changed dramatically. Marcy changed too. She emerged as the new matriarchal center of the household. When I first met her ten years earlier she was still early in her sobriety and could barely sit still. She was often abrupt. Sometimes, mid-interview, she would get up and walk out the door. She and Delores often joked that Delores was the one to run interference with the professionals (teachers, social workers, physicians) because Marcy was known to have a short fuse. But after Delores died, Marcy evinced a new authority that I had never seen. The immense sadness she felt at her mother's passing was always evident. But there was something else too—a stubborn pride, a determination that was apparent in the way she entered the room. She carried herself with dignity. "I have to do it all now," she said with a stoicism that reminded me of her mother.

Soon after Delores's death, Marcy moved the family away from Altadena, the neighborhood that Delores had called home, the place where Marcy had grown up and had longed to leave. They relocated to a town in the desert suburbs of Los Angeles where they could rent a bigger house for the same money they had been paying. Marcy thought it would be safer for the children as well. "Away from the trouble," she said. She was very hopeful about this move. It would be another beginning for them, one that she directed. Though family life had its difficulties, Leroy seemed to be doing pretty well. He was not a member of any gangs, did not do or deal drugs, performed reasonably well in school, and had ambitions to become an engineer. He was very close to Delores, and it was hard on him when she got so sick. He helped take care of her, as well as his younger siblings, especially his cousin Willy, who shared a bedroom with him. Over the years, their extended household had further expanded to include the girlfriend of Marcy's oldest son, Ralph, and their young baby. Sasha's son Willy and Marcy's children, along with Marcy's new grandson, grew up together.

In January 2008, Leroy, then sixteen, was gunned down in front of his house. Two young men in their early twenties wanted to take his younger sister for a drive. She had gotten in the backseat of their car when Leroy stormed out of the house (unarmed) and began arguing with them, protectively trying to get his sister out. "She's too young for you," he yelled. Willy went out with him and stood beside him in support. One of the men pulled out a gun and opened fire. Leroy was shot nine times. He never fell down, Marcy repeated with anguish. Staggering back into the house, he fell into his mother's arms. "Hold me Mama," he said. She held him while they waited for the ambulance. He died in the hospital two days later, after three surgeries.

I consider this event as experienced by Marcy and especially Leroy's older brother Ralph, but also by the community more broadly, through the lens of three powerful moral imaginaries: the street, the home, and the church. But it is the way spiritual discourse and authority is displayed and contested that is a focal point here. I not only examine how multiple and rival schemes become resources for debate, as in the previous chapter, but focus upon two additional resources that promote moral scrutiny: (1) the possibility to draw upon authoritative practices and discourse to level a critique of them; (2) the capability of taking a third person perspective on oneself to subject those third person categories and norms to evaluation and contestation.

In what follows, I introduce a moral space that has been in the shadows thus far—"the streets," or the public spaces of the urban poor, a place especially inhabited by young men.

"THE STREETS": LIVED EXPERIENCE AND SOCIAL IMAGINARY

Street gangs in Los Angeles remain legendary. Los Angeles is now said to be "the gang capital of the world" (The Advancement Project, 2007, p. 1). The Los Angeles Police Department (2007) recently designated the 11 most notorious gangs in the city: 18th Street Westside (Southwest Area), 204th Street (Harbor Area), Avenues (Northeast Area), Black P-Stones (Southwest, Wilshire Areas), Canoga Park Alabama (West Valley Area), Grape Street Crips (Southeast Area), La Mirada Locos (Rampart, Northeast Areas),

Mara Salvatrucha (Rampart, Hollywood, and Wilshire Areas), Rollin
40s (Southwest Area), Rollin 30s Harlem Crips (Southwest Area),
and Rolling 60s (77th St. Area).

—Howell et al, *U.S. Gang Problem Trends and Seriousness,
1996–2009, 2011*

The two cities with the most chronic gang problems, Los Angeles and
Chicago, accounted for more than half of [United States] homicides.
Also, about one in every five homicides committed in those cities
involved a gang member, and they were most likely to occur in areas
with greater populations, chronic gang presence, and a larger number
of gang members.

—Renzetti and Edleston, "Gang Violence," 2008

In Los Angeles County, law enforcement officials are aware of more
than 1300 street gangs with over 150,000 members. In the City of
Los Angeles alone, there are over 400 separate gangs and an
estimated 39,000 gang members.

—Los Angeles Mayor Antonio Villaraigosa, 2007

Los Angeles has the largest gang population in the United States, a
significant portion of which distributes illicit drugs.

—National Drug Intelligence Center 2007

Gangs account for approximately 43% of all homicides in Los Angeles
County. Of the 1038 homicides in 2004, 454 were gang-related.

—Criminal Justice Center, 2005

Los Angeles has long been recognized as the epicenter of gang
activity nationwide. Recent estimates indicate approximately 1,350
street gangs, with as many as 175,000 members in the FBI Los
Angeles' seven-county area of responsibility (San Luis Obispo, Santa
Barbara, Ventura, Los Angeles, Riverside, San Bernardino, and
Orange). Many gangs which today have a nationwide presence, such
as the Bloods, the Crips, Mara Salvatrucha (MS-13), and 18th Street
can trace their roots to Los Angeles.

—U.S. Congress, 2006

For most (over two-thirds) of the cities with populations of 50,000
or more, prevalence rates of gang activity have remained unchanged
for the past decade and a half.

—Howell et al., *U.S. Gang Problem Trends and Seriousness,
1996–2009, 2011*

Leroy's murder is all the more tragic precisely because homicides have
been so ubiquitous in the poorer areas of Los Angeles County. Although
crime rates have dropped somewhat in recent years, the threat of death,
especially for young black men, is enormous. As can be seen in the
quotes above, Los Angeles has been variously described as "the epicenter of gang activity nationwide" and "the gang capital of the world."
There have been dips and surges at times over the past three decades,

but overall the city, including some of its outlying suburbs, has continued to be an "epicenter" of gang memberships, homicide, and drug-related activity. Los Angeles represents a particularly compelling example of the demise of public life—the street not as a space of civic pride, as it once was, but of resignation and danger. When African Americans first settled in the Los Angeles area—and early migrations began in the beginning of the twentieth century—it was in answer to a dream for a better life, one in which they hoped for (and in early decades sometimes got) less racism, the possibility of buying homes, and the chance for respectable work that paid decent wages.

Communities like those that grew up around South Central, Compton, and Watts were once far more vibrant and thriving than they are today. Compare this to the situation when, according to recent 2006 figures, Compton was rated the most dangerous city in the United States, especially notorious for gang violence. The homicide rate for poor black urban areas of Los Angeles is now approximately eight times the national average. A quote from one African American writer in the 1990s documents this shift in community and street life in Los Angeles that has occurred over the past four decades:

> Talk with any Black Angelino over the age of fifty and he will wax poetic about the richness of life along Central Avenue, describing the plethora of homes, the wonderful atmosphere and music that flows from the Club Alabam and the Apex Club, the economic promise of black business ... the pride in self that sprung from the bookstores, literary guilds, and community organizations like the YMCA or Gavery's UNIA. Compare that passion with the spirit of resignation that accompanies his discussion about life along "the avenue" in 1989. (Bunch 1990:123, cited in Jacobs 2000:39)

"The streets" is a moral space associated with urban poverty—a synonym for the ghetto. While to be "street" marks a kind of virtuosity, showing quickness and adeptness at navigating socially and a mastery of urban street culture, it also symbolizes a way of life characterized by hustling, getting ahead at the expense of anyone else, and a tough willingness to do whatever it takes for financial gain. It has characteristically been far more closely associated with the activities and identity formation of African American men than women. Some contend that especially for marginalized African American men, "'the streets' is a socialization institution that is as important as the family, the church, and the educational system" (Oliver 2006: 919).[1] Exclusion from mainstream forms of employment and upward mobility has helped to make the streets an attractive place for young African American men to combat a sense of invisibility and marginalization, offering a central space to achieve social status.[2]

"The streets" figures as a central moral imaginary that has helped to produce a portrait of underclass black male identity in stereotypical ways (e.g., hypersexual, aggressive, dangerous, irresponsible), including being "absent fathers."[3] The streets and the African American man have become intertwined cultural figures in American popular culture. African American scholars have critiqued this portrayal, fueled by the media, especially in its depiction of African American men as, variously, "gangster rappers, hustlers, rapists, gang bangers, drug dealers, crack heads."[4]

Wacquant cautions, "One must guard against the confused and confusing invocation of notions, like that of 'ghetto', that operate as mere metaphors calling forth an emotive imagery that hides fundamental structural and functional differences, thereby stopping inquiry just where it should get going" (2008:8). The structural features Wacquant refers to are readily apparent in Los Angeles. The ubiquity of guns, the prevalence of gangs, the attraction of the drug trade as a primary means of employment among youth disenfranchised by race and class from other economic possibilities, the continued abandonment of the poor in America, the surging private prison business (and the fact that much of the drug business is run from prisons), the disproportionate incarceration of African Americans—all these conspire to create a dangerous situation. The vast underemployment of African American men, twice that of whites (a problem intensified by the demise of so much of the blue-collar industry in Los Angeles) has been a very significant factor in this.[5]

The government has also played a key role. Its policies reflect an exaggeration of the drug trade among poor African Americans that has helped mobilize a harsh punitive policy response that targets black Americans.[6] The most visible state-directed form of control is the police. Well before the introduction of street drugs and the rise of violent gangs (which grew rapidly in the 1980s), police have been a force of state control in black urban street life that has generated outrage in the community. Police tactics have been particularly ferocious against its young men. Though contentious relationships between police and African Americans is an old American story,[7] it has had a particularly public face in Los Angeles. The Watts uprisings of 1965 and the riots surrounding the police beating of Rodney King in 1992 are just two examples of the problematic relationships between police and black Angelinos that are well remembered in the Los Angeles African American community.

These interlinked political, racial, and economic factors have created an urban environment in which gang violence and a lethal drug industry have come to dominate the public space. Gang-related violence is not confined to gang members, however, and is not primarily related to drug transactions. Much of it is triggered by neighborhood turf battles or threats to social status. There are literally hundreds of gangs in Los Angeles. Each gang tries to hold control over particular neighborhoods, and these can be up for dispute.[8] Challenges to neighborhood control can instigate a spate of violence. To be out on the street in an unfamiliar neighborhood as a young African American male can be dangerous business indeed. Marcy wondered whether her decision to move the family to a new neighborhood had left Leroy unprotected. The streets in her old neighborhood were dangerous, but at least her boys were known by the surrounding gangs, especially her oldest son Ralph, a member of the local Bloods, one of LA's largest and most powerful gangs.

HOME AS SANCTUARY FROM THE STREETS

Marcy's sense of moral failure reveals one of the most difficult tasks that parents in underclass neighborhoods are compelled to take on: creating homes that can serve as physical and moral sanctuaries from the streets. "The streets" were often experienced by parents in our study as a land of danger, violence, lawlessness, where the prevalence of drugs and guns represent constant threats to the safety of their children and themselves. The police were not trusted and were often perceived as not only unhelpful but an active source of danger. Children were kept inside the house as much as possible, especially after dark. As these parents have pointed out repeatedly, an enormous part of their work is devoted to what constitutes being a "good" parent: keeping their children safe from the streets. In chapter 3, Delores "rescues" Marcy from the street, and a large part of that rescue not only means, quite literally, bringing her home, but also *creating* home on an everyday basis. Even among families like Delores's where dealing drugs has, at least at times, been a primary way to make a living (in this case, for Sasha, Marcy, and Ralph), the spaces of home and street are not only depicted as geographically distinct but, most important, as ethically differentiated. They operate according to different local moralities.

There are certain heroic tales that family members have told about protecting a child from street violence even at the risk of their own lives. One of the women in our study described a day when her son was out with her own mother and they had stopped at a gas station. As her son was walking into the station, a man came up and put a gun to his head, saying his brother had just gotten killed and he was out for revenge. The grandmother got out of the car and went right up and hugged the man. He broke down and started crying and then he apologized. This small, poignant tale underscores not only the prevalence of violence but also the tragedy of its randomness and the humanity of the perpetrator, one who also suffers, who is also a victim of violence.

Parents try to create homes that are fortresses of a kind, ones that can be insulated, as far as possible, against the danger of an outside urban world. But these are fragile fortresses. Andrew and Darlene (the parents in the previous chapter), for example, built a fence on their rental property in an effort to keep children in and street life out. However, one day the street brutally intruded. The family became victims of armed robbery, as Darlene put it. She and Andrew co-narrated the event. "Two men with guns did a home invasion on us," Darlene reported. "They pushed us in our house and pulled guns on me, my husband and my children. . . . One guy hit me [with the gun] . . . and then the same guy hit my husband also." As a result, and on the advice of the police, Andrew and Darlene moved away from the South Central neighborhood they had known their whole lives. Andrew said, "The officers told us it'd be a good thing to move because one of the guys is still at large. And he done killed somebody else since we been left." They rented a house in one of the high-desert community towns surrounding Los Angeles that had affordable (Section 8) housing, but it was a two-hour commute from their old neighborhood, friends, and church.

Cherishing small family routines and jokes ("Who stole the TV remote?" "Grandma, this tastes like dog food!") makes a special kind of sense when contrasted with the dramatic dangers posed just outside the front door—perhaps even in the front yard or inside the house when a home invasion occurs. Andrew and Darlene succeeded in moving their children out of the neighborhood and no one was hurt. Delores succeeded in rescuing Marcy. But Marcy was not so fortunate. She did not save her boy from harm. Is she to blame? she wonders. Despite her efforts to take her mother's place and to remain sober for so many years, perhaps she is not yet wise enough to protect her own children. A few days after the funeral she remarked, her ordinarily boisterous voice soft with remorse, that Delores, who had had twelve children, "never lost any of them." Only two months after her mother's death, she had already lost one of her sons.

THE CHURCH AND THE STREET IN DIALOGUE

In Los Angeles, federal, state, and city authorities continue to look primarily at stricter punishments and prison sentences for violent offenders. But at a local neighborhood level, from inside the community, people explore other options. At both a neighborhood park memorial and a funeral service for Leroy, participants draw upon a discourse of personal confession to invoke both an indigenous "hermeneutics of critique" and a "hermeneutics of hope" surrounding this violence. The street is contrasted with the spiritual—with the authority of God and the institution of the church.[9] Not only confessing sinners but also the community and the Christian church come under moral scrutiny. The street emerges not merely as a negative moral space but also as having a moral potentiality and authority that neither home nor church possesses. In describing the park memorial and the church service, I consider four cultural vehicles that participants draw upon. Two of these resources will now be familiar: the creation of moral laboratories in everyday spaces and the use of one authoritative moral discourse to critique an alternative moral discourse. I highlight two additional resources I have not yet fully discussed. One is the explicit and self-conscious use of one's assigned (third person) subject position to critique the moral normativity surrounding that position. Another is the use of authoritative cultural tools (in this case, confession) to challenge moral authority—a form of challenge from within a single moral "regime of truth."

I have insisted that it is important to consider moral experimentation of the everyday without reducing it to a simple resistance theory of agency or presuming that actors are primarily moved by political concerns. But the political is often not far from sight. Although this might be expressed as a mode of resistance, it is also expressed in the language of natality, in the effort to bring something new into personal and public being. Already with Tanya, the first parent I introduced, we can see that her efforts to care for her intimate others, her son and her family, led her into increasingly political and public battles. She tells us, although with a little embarrassment that she might sound too grand, that she is engaging in a form of revolution. The event that follows Leroy's death most closely reveals a relationship between the moral and the frankly political, even the revolutionary. The need for something like revolution is voiced through the protests, confessions, and invocations that arise.

RALPH'S CONFESSION: THE NEIGHBORHOOD PARK AS MORAL LABORATORY

I offer a few lines from the lament spoken by Ralph, Leroy's older brother, a man in his late twenties. He speaks at a candlelight vigil just three days before Leroy's funeral and two days after Leroy died in the hospital. This gathering of friends, families, and neighbors takes place in a small, shabby park central to the black section of his home town (a township within Los Angeles County and a few miles from the city itself). As usual, the park is populated with locals involved in numerous drug exchanges or in drinking, talking, laughing, flirting, smoking. The mourners simply ignore this activity as they walk solemnly holding candles, to gather in a circle around Ralph. Family members protectively surround Olga, the researcher who filmed the vigil. Leroy's mother Marcy cautions a friend, "I'm gonna stand with her. She don't want nobody to trip on her cause she videotaping. They don't know who she is." Leroy's family wants this moment documented, and his mother directs friends to let others in the park know that Olga is videotaping by request. Participants in the vigil take the candles they have lit and place them on the ground near Ralph, at the center of the circle they have formed.

Though many people will speak at the funeral, at this vigil Ralph is the only speaker. His words are addressed less to the women and children in the crowd than to the young men gathered, men who, like himself, have been (or are) in gangs and have lived with violence. He speaks in a tone so angry and sad, so broken, that his words are difficult to listen to. His words, which at first seem fragmented, a torrent of despair, were, as I realized upon listening more carefully, a melody of rage and blame as well as a ferocious plea.

It is sometimes argued that when great pain happens, there are no words to express it. There is a truth to that. But it is also true that poetry can arise at such moments, aesthetic creations that seem to be born from suffering itself. And so, in the face of the unjust death of his brother, Ralph abandons the casualness of ordinary speech. Instead, he offers a spontaneous prose poem, a hip-hop directive to the community to end the deaths and the killing. I have organized his words into stanzas to highlight the poetry of his language, the rhythms that bear down on the audience, so that even if—as he insists—no one understands, no one listens, he will speak, he will plead, he will confess, he will say the unsayable, he will say what must be said:

I die.
My momma dies.
Everybody dies niggah.
My grandma died.
Ya'll don't know homie.
All this shit, God, is fucked up niggah.
We started the police trippin on us niggah.
Ya'll did it niggah, that's why ya'll gettin it hard niggah.
We did it.
[I'm] one of the first niggah's on probation for gang shit, niggah.
Ya'll don't understand niggah.
They got us in a trap niggah.
I've been in prison, back, everywhere.
Ya'll going there too, keep doing that homie.
I'm telling you.
This shit fucked up.
Ya'll don't understand homie.

Ralph begins to cry as he continues his anguished rap.

Ya'll don't understand homie.
No.
Man, my little brother, man I got to deal with this thing all in my sleep
*   and everything.*
That's fucked up.
Sixteen.
No hope niggah.

Ralph shifts from this general lament and indictment of black–on–black violence to a graphic narration of the murder. He punctuates his narration with an enactment of where the bullets entered Leroy's body, pointing to his own body to illustrate. If these "homies" refuse to understand, he will compel their understanding, making them *feel* the entrance of the bullets, one by one. And he will admonish them to listen to their mothers and their grandmothers, to do whatever it takes to keep themselves safe.

Ya'll gonna keep doing that stupid shit.
And it took for my little brother to get shot for me to understand that
*   this shit is not stupid.*
It's not a game or nothin' homie.
Ya'll got to understand this.
Please understand this.
I'm asking ya'll niggah.
I don't ask people "please."
I don't say "please homie," unless I really want you to do it.
Please don't do that homie.

He got shot nine times, niggah.
Seven of the bullets stayed in his body, two of em went out.
He fought.
Ya'll got a lot to learn man.
All that shit we been through, it ain't nothin man.
He fought on the [operating] table.
He, he, got hit niggah nine times.
Five times right here. (Ralph points towards his chest.)
Bam.
Five times. One time right here. (Ralph points toward his wrist.)
The niggah was running, he got hit in his ass niggah. (Ralph points to his buttocks.)
He tried to get in the house, he got hit in his fucking liver.
One shot is all it took.
Liver, lungs, all that shit that's in your stomach.
One bullet hit that Leroy, and went in there. (Points to stomach.)
You know why that happened?
Cause he ran.
He kept moving.
If he would've stayed still he probably would've lived.
He ran in the house, sat on the fucking couch man.

He fought hard.
He had three surgeries man.
He had three surgeries homie.
I don't know what it feel like to have no surgery.
He had three of 'em.
He went through all the surgeries.
They told us he was doing good.
His heart started going down homie.
He just stopped fucking pumpin.
It slowly stopped pumping homie.

Ralph concludes the story of his brother's death by returning to his admonition to the crowd (and to himself) that black street violence has got to stop. For him, what emerges as especially unbearable is that his brother was an innocent victim. He wasn't meant for the streets. He was planning to become an engineer. Even white people cared about him, Ralph said. He was afraid to shoot a gun. He wasn't meant to be the one who got killed. Maybe Ralph and others might die—they lived by violence—but "Leroy wasn't with that."

Tellin ya'll, this is with all ya'll man.
Ya'll know Leroy wasn't with that.
And he felt it. [The pain of violence.]
You know what I'm sayin?

It's some of, you niggahs didn't even feel it, but Leroy did homie.
That's how life go. God show us. You know what I'm saying.
Better than he can tell us.
And he tired of tellin us.
He gonna keep showin us and showin us and showin us until we get it
  right.
Look what that say niggah.

(Ralph points to a sign someone holds up high for everyone to see. It reads "WE MUST STOP KILLING US!")

All you niggahs have probably seen this black car driving down the
  street with that (Referring to the sign) *on the side of the car niggah.*
All you niggahs homie, been seeing that sign right there.
Niggah drive up and down the street in that black car.
And he serious.
We must stop killing us.
Two black niggahs just killed Leroy, another black niggah.
And now we right here, I've gotta talk to ya'll.
Leroy wasn't half of the things that some of us was homie.
You know that.
He wasn't even thinking about none of that stuff.
Niggah, Leroy wanted to be an engineer homie.
Ya'll don't even know the white people that came to my house that day
  niggah. [After Leroy died]
(Starting to sob) *Gave cards for my man.*
I fucked up homie!

Ralph breaks down, crying hard. He walks over to a man in the crowd and they put their arms around each other. He calls out to the crowd one last time:

Fucked up my brother!

And with this, the vigil ends.

Ralph's lament is not merely a piece of spontaneous poetry, not merely an expression of a quintessentially African American cultural form. It is that and it is something else besides. It is a form of moral deliberation. Ralph's lament raises such questions as, Who is to blame? Who can fix things? What can be hoped for? What can be done? How can this be bearable? What do we have to learn here? What have we not understood? What is required of us? How were we not just doing wrong but *seeing* wrong? What is it about our values and practices that leads us to this blindness? Why must we blame ourselves and not God, not even the "theys" who trap the disempowered?

The pondering over who is to blame is not, of course, a factual consideration (notably, he never lays blame directly on the young man who shot Leroy) but an ethical one. It is bound up not only with despair but also with hope because it is about the possibility of agency, of social change. Ralph tells them, only in coming to see more rightly, more wisely, will the community of "homies," his community, have any agency in turning the violence around. He lays blame to present lessons, where he sees that something can and must be learned. Here, many are culpable—Leroy and those who do not listen to their "mamas." Himself for "fucking up." The "they" of authorities, of a (white) social structure that "got us in a trap." More pervasively, the community of "homies" and "niggahs" who, like himself, have been blind, refused to understand that violence is not "stupid." *Stupid* is too insipid a word for it. *Stupid* refuses the depth of despair that a truer, wiser gaze reveals. Violence is "not a game" but something much more heartbreaking. It must, at all costs, be stopped. "WE MUST STOP KILLING US!" he reads as a mourner holds up the sign high above his head for all the crowd to see.

Ralph is "becoming a sinner" in a heightened way (Robbins 2004). And he exhorts his listeners to do likewise. He levels an unrelenting critical gaze on his own blindness and moral weakness, even though he was not culpable in any direct way. Confession is bound up not only with critique but also with hope because it is about the possibility of social change. In his challenge, he juxtaposes the ethics of the streets with a rival Christian ethics and a God who insists on "showing us and showing us" the sinfulness of this street life through such tragedies as the death of his innocent brother.

In the park Ralph's confession performs what, to paraphrase Kenneth Burke (1945), one might call "scenic violations." The "streets" become a momentary street church in Ralph's lament. Ralph uses his street-style confession to challenge the street life in which he has been a major participant. And he uses a street forum, this neighborhood park, as a space of critique, transforming it into a temporary "moral laboratory" in which an ordinary space for dealing drugs becomes a space for decrying this very life. Through Ralph's anguished poetry, and through the respectful listening of the gathered crowd, the park is transformed into a space of possibility.

THE STREETS AS MORAL RESOURCE

Leroy's funeral was held at a local church in the old neighborhood of Altadena where Marcy had grown up and where Leroy and his family lived most of their lives. As the service starts, every seat is taken and the pulpit is crowded with ministerial staff. Along the outside walls surrounding the seated congregation stand young men dressed in red, the Blood's gang colors. They have filed in silently, gracefully, in full uniform. I thought of soldiers coming to pay their respects to one of their own fallen. Leroy was not theirs, but still, they could come to show support to his devastated brother Ralph, who very much was.

After several songs and formal sermons by the ministers, members from the congregation to stood up to speak. One of them was Ralph, here again directing his attention to fellow gang members, the young men who lined the back of the church. "We have got to stop the killing," he repeated again and again. "This world is a cold, cruel place," Leroy's best friend said in a poem she wrote and read aloud at the service. The minister tried to reassure the audience that Leroy was just "on loan" and he was now in a better place, but the misery in the room was palpable. Even the praise hymns sounded anguished. Yet, the response of families like Leroy's does not reflect the resigned despair that Daniel Valentine (1996) documents among the Sri Lankans, or that Scheper-Hughes (1993) observes among destitute Brazilian mothers who have come to accept the inevitable deaths of children "without weeping." Instead, such despair is resisted, fought against. Leroy's extended family struggles to find ways for his death to serve as a mode of "witness," to call out to others in the community to "stop the killing."

But "resistance" is not quite an accurate description of what Ralph is doing. We can hear this in what Ralph says when he stands up at the funeral. He has turned to face family and friends (especially his uncle and fellow gang members) who have been part of the very violence that must be stopped. He speaks in a tone quite different from his park lament. He has dropped street vernacular, but still he insists, yet again, that people (outsiders) "might be watching" (or judging) but "they don't know." What they don't know is that something must happen from inside the community, from "on the inside," from the street itself. If the street is a resource, this is because those living this life are the ones whose desire for change is most palpable. Ralph speaks only after his own uncle, himself once a gang member, has spoken in bitter rage, proclaiming that those who hurt his family ought to be punished. Ralph offers a contrasting message, half-turning to his still standing uncle so that his words speak both to him personally as well as fellow gang members collectively. Ralph invokes the first person plural here to challenge his uncle and to redirect the moral energy of this "we."

We gotta step up, I'm telling you.
We got to step up homie.
If we don't step up for him [Leroy], it's gonna be over.
I'm telling you, they too young.
It's people that just watching us.
But they don't know.
It's people like you and me that wanna change it.
But they won't help us homie.

Hope and despair sound nearly the same here. Why should one hope? Because one can't afford the luxury of despair. All of the "theys"—the government, the middle class, whites, power authorities, in fact, everyone who is not part of street life—nothing can be expected from them. "They won't help us homie." Only homies can help, not because they have more resources but because the alternative is unthinkable. "If we don't step up," Ralph says, "it's gonna be over." The "it" that will be over is moral life. Things have gone too far. "I'm telling you, they too young." Ralph's only hope is grounded in the sense that the moral violation is now so thorough that people like him are ready to do something. "It may not look like it on the outside, but on the inside it's a lot of people around here that talk about changing it," he says. But he offers no optimism here. There is no miraculous conversion available—just very hard human effort. He concludes, in a poetic refrain that recalls his opening admonition that "we gotta step up."

But this, man, it takes time.
It takes stairs.
We at a low pole.
We just want the younger ones to get it right

CRITIQUE AND EXPERIMENT WITHIN A TRADITION: THE PRAYER WARRIOR CONFESSES IN CHURCH

Ralph is not the only one that day to offer a funeral address that basically states that it is going to be up to "homies" to transform the violent street because no one else knows or cares enough. A young woman also brings this message to the listening congregation. But she introduces a new interpretation that reframes Ralph's point. Ralph's words are primarily directed to his fellow homies. When he invokes the spiritual, as he does in his park lament, it is the street that is to be scrutinized critically in light of the spiritual. However, this young woman has something different to say. She is dressed neither in "church" clothes as many are, nor in gang clothes as others are, but more casually, in jeans. Her fiery challenge is to the church as an authority. It is this moral space that she brings under scrutiny. The ministers and the "good" churchgoers, as she depicts them, turn out to be, if not exactly sinners, at least guilty of having turned their backs on their own children and their community.

She begins by speaking in an intimate way to Marcy, who is sitting in the front row. She notes, her own voice shaking, that she too has recently lost someone dear through street violence. She then shifts tone. She declares, her voice growing stronger and angrier, that although she is a believer, she is also a warrior. She herself has come from the streets, come from fighting, and this experience has taught her "it's not about coming to church. It's about the church going into the streets for the lost, and for the broken, and for the world."

Her voice rises as she speaks, and the congregation claps at her fiery words. She continues, fiercer in her declarations, her cadence ever more rhythmic, drawing words that fuse the poetry of street rap, church testimonials, and hymns.

> *Everybody don't know and don't understand.*
> *You have to come out of the building.*
> *We have to hit the streets.*
> *We have to get down like that.*
> *That's this time that's for this generation.*

The congregation claps harder, listening as she gains momentum, sounding like the warrior she has declared herself to be, a soldier in a revolution that God is leading.

> *That's what it's gonna take.*
> *It's gonna take us to come out.*
> *It's gonna take us to be soldiers of God.*
> *That's how much I believe God.*
> *I believe God about to strike up out of this building.*
> *And [I] do what I have to do as a woman of God.*
> *(Congregation claps)*
> *Save, deliver and change!*

Directing her gaze to the young men lining the walls of the church, she continues:

> *It ain't gonna take a funeral for y'all to be comin'.*
> *No!*

Then turning to ministers on the front stage and the congregation at large:

We need to be out here.
To be hittin' the streets and talkin' to the people and mentor them about
  God!

She then confesses her own sinfulness, her life as a "gangsta," as evidence that her exhortations to "come out of the church" to the streets have merit.

God didn't save me [in a church].
I came from the hood.
I was a gangsta.
I shot and I did all of that.
Don't be mistaken 'cause I'm a female.
(Someone in the congregation calls "That's right.")
I got down where I was mad at everyone.
Now I'm sayin' God turned me around, how much more can he do it
  for y'all? (Congregation claps.)
How much more can he do it for y'all?
But I believe.
I'm a believer.

She exhorts the congregation and the ministers yet again.

We need to get out there.
We need to let them know that we care.
We need to let them know that we love them.
Why?
'Cause God loves us.

Her final words are to Ralph as she promises that she will not leave him in the streets by himself. If he is going to return to the streets, she will be there too.

I love you Ralph.
I told you, "When I see you in the streets, I'll be right there too.
And let you know I'm there."
'Cause I have God in my heart.
And it ain't no hood love.
It's God's love.
(Congregation claps resoundingly as she walks back to her seat.)

While the ministers in the pulpit address the sinners (especially the young men lining the walls of the church), she primarily addresses the ministers. And she uses confession, a central discourse of the institution, as a vehicle for making her challenge. Her very sinfulness, her past history, gives her the authority to critique the pious, the ministers, those who stay safe inside the sanctuary. She demands that the safely saved rethink how to be a church. She asks what such a sacred community is responsible to do, what its moral mission is in these hard times when children are dying every day.

Her final promise to Ralph furthers this challenge. Is it only her, the prayer warrior, who will be with him? Or is she also saying something about God's presence in the streets? Is it God, having "struck out of the building," who will be with him even if he returns to his life in the streets? And is this ambiguity a way of marking that there is a deep flaw in an older generation of Christians who continue to insist that one must come to church to be saved, thereby abandoning "the lost," "the broken," even "the world"?

DUELING CONFESSIONS AS DIALOGICAL POSSIBILITY

Through the prayer warrior's challenge to the church, turning confession against itself, so to speak, she brings the streets into the church. She turns the church into a moral laboratory, an experimental glimpse of another kind of church not confined to its walls. And she does something else as well. Although she rarely directs herself overtly to those lining the walls, standing silently together in their gang colors, her confession of who she has been and where she has come from speaks to a possible self that they too might become. Like her, they might become a different kind of warrior, prayer warriors dedicated to a higher calling than (so she implies) even the ministers at the pulpit offer.

If she is able to draw upon a tradition of confession and her own position as a (former) sinner, this is possible in large part because of the special role the African American church has had in the black community. Institutionally, African American churches have developed with a distinctive mission that leave them open for distinctive kinds of political and moral challenge.[10] The church's technologies of ethical self-making (like public confession) can be mobilized against its own authority precisely because the African American church has historically intertwined a political mission with a spiritual one. I mentioned this briefly in the previous chapter but it bears elaborating here where the church is not only a source of authority but also a target of critique.

It is widely recognized that the black church has been the single most important institution for mounting efforts at social, political, and economic change for poor African Americans.[11] Churches have provided all kinds of practical supports—childcare facilities, schools, even low-income housing, banks, and insurance companies, and health care programs.[12]Local neighborhood churches have provided primary social communities for making friends, sharing personal concerns, and creating a wider network outside one's family. Within the African American church, spirituality and healing can carry political messages—in fact, the idea of "healing" within this religious vocabulary readily speaks to social problems.[13] Sometimes this religious discourse has been directed to the wider national public, as in fights for civil rights. But in many cases it has also been activist in less resistance-based manner, providing social support to its members or surrounding neighborhoods—especially targeting the community's poor.

Pastors of black churches have often seen their roles as including overseeing this wide range of support services. They are likely to explain their willingness to bring their churches into active cooperation with social programs based on taking a "holistic" approach to their work—recognizing that the spiritual is bound up with all manner of other practical and earthly concerns.[14] The spiritual, communal, practical, political, and aesthetic are fused in a single social institution.[15] The economic conditions in which black urban churches, in particular, emerged after large numbers of African Americans moved from the South into major urban centers during the Great Migration (from 1914 to 1922) also created a visible and local street presence.[16] If this extension of the church into the everyday lives of the community, and especially of the poor, endangered, and disenfranchised, has been part of its moral purpose, this also leaves the church open to criticism. What the prayer warrior's words show is the way spiritual discourse can be harnessed for political purposes, to enable debate and mobilize a conversation within the African American community. Her confessional challenge also echoes a sentiment sometimes voiced within the African American religious community more broadly, where there has been debate over the abandonment of the church's traditional social responsibilities to poor communities.[17]

The Counter-Confession

The ministers who she seems particularly keen to address are vulnerable to her confession in light of their pastoral responsibility of social advocacy. How do they respond to her challenge? The presiding minister mounts a defense—notably, with a confession of his own. He announces to the congregation that he doesn't usually give his own personal testimony but he will do so today. Through his counter-confession, a confession that offers an oppositional moral position to the one the prayer warrior gives, the space of the church becomes a place to consider and reconsider its moral role vis-à-vis the dangers of the street and the vulnerability of its young men. He opens with these lines:

> God got some folk that are delivered in the church. God got some folk that came out of dope in the church. Got some anointed folk in the church. There's nothin' wrong with God's church. Amen! Hallelujah! I don't tell my testimony much, but I'm gonna tell it today, hallelujah! The devil is a lie. Hallelujah! The devil is a lie.

He tells the congregation that he is very familiar with the streets. He once belonged to them. He "burned" himself there. His confession is delivered with a powerful poetic rhythm, a rhetorical *tour de force* that rivets the audience.

> *Fourteen years, shootin' dope in my arm.*
> *Fourteen years, shootin' cocaine in my vein.*
> *Fourteen years, smokin' crack.*
> *Burned myself on Skid Row.*
> *Sleepin' on the streets.*
> *The devil is a lie,*
> *God got folk in the church that will deliver you.*
> *God got folk in the church.*

He pauses to let people cheer and clap. Some call out in enthusiastic support, although the young men lining the walls are unmoved. As members of the seated congregation become increasingly stirred by his words, his voice and demeanor intensify. He adds details of place and time in a vivid rendering of his own rescue.

> Found myself on Skid Row. Downtown 5th street. Sleepin' on the street. I wanted to go into a program. They told me, "We don't take folk like that. We only take folk at 5 in the mornin'. And you got to be the first one at the door." Amen. I wanted to be delivered. Didn't nobody come to me. I went to, to where I needed to be, hallelujah! I laid there on the ground until five in the morning. I saw the rats run by. I laid there, 'cause I made up in my mind that I wanted to be delivered, hallelujah! When they opened the door at five in the mornin', I just rolled in, hallelujah! Somebody give my God some praise! (Pause for cheering.) When I got to the church, when I got to the church, the doors was open. When I got to the church, the lights was on. When I got to the church, they had a man, named Bishop Grant Simpson, that knew what I needed for my deliverance. Brought me out, hallelujah! The devil is a lie, ain't nothin' wrong with the church!

He moves into the concluding passage of his testimony by repeating his key refrain, one that sums up his rebuttal succinctly: "Ain't nothin' wrong with the church." He has drawn upon his own first person authority as someone familiar with sin as evidence for the truth of what he claims. His rousing confession has captivated many. Some have stood up to show that they have heard his message.

> Hallelujah! Hallelujah! Somebody give God the highest praise! Hallelujah! Hallelujah! I ain't ashamed of where I come from. Because I know where I'm going—Hallelujah!—I'm not ashamed of what I went through. Cuz I'm gonna use it to beat against the gates of hell. Let my brother go, let my brother go. Loosen my children, in the name of Jesus. Somebody give God a praise in here!

Half the congregation are now on their feet, clapping as he reiterates his primary argument one last time.

> You don't see fourteen years of dope when you see me, 'cause I don't bear the image of it. What you see on me, is what my Lord sent from heaven. What you see on me is the image of living God. What you see on me is where I'm going, not where I been. Somebody gonna give God a praise in this house?

Having powerfully addressed his challenger, he returns to a traditional ending to the ceremony with a call to members of the audience to come to the altar and be saved.

> And if you love the Lord it will make you get up out of your seat and say, "You know what? Not another day. Not another day." *(Congregation claps, as people approach the stage)* "Not another day. Not another day. I'm comin' to you Lord, not another day. I'm not going to sit unregenerated. Not one more day. Not one more day. Not one more day. Not one more day."

INDIGENOUS SOURCES OF CRITIQUE AND HOPE

Leroy's death calls three social spaces into scrutiny: the home (as embodied in Marcy as Superstrong Black Mother and Ralph, an Otherfather who should keep children safe), the street, and the church. In the very promise of its moral reach, in the hope that is invested in it, the church offers resources for its own critique. In its failure to keep a young man safe, it is exposed. And, paradoxically, the streets, the very source of danger, may be the space from which hope must come. In the prayer warrior's confession, she suggests that one cannot even look to this sacred home grown institution—the African American church—for protection. Neither her condemnation of the church nor Ralph's of the street are intended to voice despair. This is precisely the response that both Ralph and the prayer warrior reject, and reject in the strongest possible terms. Even if one is to blame (as Ralph believes himself to be), that is not reason for surrender, to accept one's fate passively.

FIRST PERSON CRITIQUES OF THIRD PERSON SELVES

I conclude by mentioning, briefly, another resource for challenge, the ability to mount a challenge upon a normative discourse and subject position by critically juxtaposing one's (first person) lived experience with those normative ideals. Both the prayer warrior's and the minister's addresses to the congregation suggest that this resource is of special importance in illuminating how the moral ordinary can offer spaces for its own critical appraisal. Explicitly naming oneself from a certain third person perspective—calling attention to how one is recognized in a way that judges and condemns—can be used to protest the very norms that inform those condemnations. The prayer warrior identifies herself as a former gangsta, someone society (presumably including members of the church audience) categorizes as sinful, dangerous, criminal. From the way she proclaims this, it becomes clear that her purpose here is not so much to condemn her former life as to refute those who would abandon her and those like her, who would misrecognize her, who would be blinded to her moral possibilities, her capability for love and goodness, her calling to a moral mission.

There may be resources for critique and challenge but they certainly do not guarantee success. When the minister provides a counter-challenge, his words also stir the congregation—they have clear persuasive power. Notably, he calls upon this same resource. He, too, uses a first person narrative and position to challenge a third person identity. He identifies himself in his former life, as a drug addict. He tells the congregation that prior to dragging himself into the church, he was someone who lived on 5th Street, an area of Central Los Angeles notorious for its homeless population. (Marcy was taken to this area by a drug counselor so that she could see what she would face if her addiction continued.) The minister announces dramatically that he was living in a place of lost souls where only the most hardcore crack and heroin addicts have resided. That he has come from this place and identity to a revered spot in front of the pulpit—able to command the attention of an entire room—enacts his counter-argument. If he can do this, a once-upon-a-time addict, then he has not only proclaimed that others can also do it—against the statistics—but also that this is the way that the church reaches out to those in need. Notably, in his narrative, he tells us that when he initially tries to get into the church he is, in fact, turned away and told to come back at five in the morning. And this is what he does.

In his confession, he is countering the prayer warrior's accusation *not* by saying that the church lacks a responsibility to the poor or to those on drugs. His life offers a living testimony that God, through the church, does take responsibility and that the church can and does help even the most destitute and downtrodden. If only they take the first step. He adroitly simultaneously critiques one version of the subject position of the homeless black crack and heroin addict (someone viewed as morally irredeemable) and defends the authority of the church. Since he, quite literally, occupies center stage standing at his pulpit, he is able to have the last word.

CHAPTER 9

Tragedy, Possibility, and Philosophical Anthropology

It is a tricky business to speak of moral possibility when considering a group of people as systematically disenfranchised as those I have written about. I have filled this book with tragic tales. These tragedies not only document a relentless onslaught of bad luck and the structural oppression that poverty and racism deliver. They also reveal how deeply people find themselves haunted by the possibility of moral failure, by their inability to sufficiently protect the vulnerable children in their care, or to protect their own moral hearts. And yet, this is not a despairing book. In considering the moral efforts and ground projects of families whose lives I have recounted, I have found myself compelled to think against a certain kind of suspicion.

A skeptical ethos has long dominated social and philosophical thought. Ricoeur has referred to it as a "hermeneutics of suspicion" (1981:113) and Charles Taylor has described it as a growing "moral imagination of unbelief" that arose in the nineteenth century and continues to thrive (2007:369). As part of this ethos, new kinds of critiques of personal and social life became possible. New insights were put forward that revealed the immense propensity of humans to be mystified about the circumstances of their lives, to operate with false categories and assumptions. The great intellectual projects dedicated to uncovering and revealing this human capacity to be misled—believing things about oneself and the world that are untrue, or (in its most radical rendition) believing that there are truths when there is only, as Nietzsche put it, a "mobile army of metaphors"—have been enormously fruitful. Exercises that debunk or destabilize the most basic truisms of (Western) common sense continue to inspire social theory. The poststructural influence and postmodern thought have enormously furthered this mistrustful gaze. One could say that we contemporary social theorists have collectively become masters of suspicion.

Many insights have been generated by these skeptical proposals, including those in a posthumanist vein that ask us to reimagine our concept of the human altogether. Nevertheless, they can come with serious costs. In particular, the complexities of motive, of moral deliberation and moral creativity as elements of ordinary life, are difficult to discern or are even dismissed altogether. I have asked (implicitly): Can't we critique modernity's moral universalisms and Eurocentric common sense without completely devaluing notions of agency, personhood, experience, biographical selves, interpretive self-reflection, and the like—thereby throwing the baby out with the bathwater? Without a strong theory of the human subject as a complex moral agent capable of *acting upon history* (even if within a history that also makes her) as well as an agent compelled to *respond* to history, including the small histories that comprise ordinary life, then we, as scholars, miss a great deal about how social life takes shape, what morally matters to people, and even how social change might occur.

On analogous lines, if the moral ordinary does not afford us resources for critique and transformation, then social change can only come about through radical breaches from the ordinary—for example, "limit experiences," historical revolutions, and other forms of dramatic discontinuities—or by heroic transgressive figures and movements. Although transgressive historical moments, movements, and experiences are undoubtedly important in shaping new moral possibilities and should not be underestimated, there is the worrisome possibility of either nihilistic skepticism (who can predict a revolution that will offer new possibilities?) or romantic elitism (few have the courage to speak the truth in Socratic fashion, after all). I have argued that it is more promising to consider the moral ordinary from the vantage point of its potentialities as well as its repressive normativities.

The first person virtue ethics I have proposed presumes that ordinary people under ordinary conditions face complex moral situations that demand our analytic attention. To elucidate this, I have drawn upon an ancient philosophical tradition that portrays practical action as a vulnerable ethical drama. I turned initially to Aristotle's theory of praxis that makes a moral (and vulnerable) agent central and the search for a "situated good" as well as the cultivation of moral virtues a primary practical task. My dramatistic portrait considers the temporal complexity of moral becoming, its rootedness in past histories as well as its link to possible futures. But it is not about good people as opposed to, say, evil ones. To return to a point made in the opening chapters and persuasively put forward by a number of anthropologists, taking morality seriously does not presume that people are good but rather that they are evaluative in moral terms about their own actions and those of others, (cf. Lambek 2010a; Laidlaw 2013; Read 1955; Robbins 2013).

The ground project I have attended to is care of intimate others in the context of family life. The first person I foreground is an inextricably relational one, bound up not only within the communal "we" of families and other social networks but charged with the care of others (the second person perspective is implicit), morally intertwined with them, compelled to respond even in situations of estrangement. I have relied on the notion of "responsivity" as explicitly developed by some phenomenologists (Wentzer, 2014) and more implicitly argued in virtue ethics. I have written primarily about five families, returning again and again to Delores's extended household to consider the vagaries of moral experience and the shifting projects of moral transformation undertaken by various family members. While I have often foregrounded women in this book, as well as the subject position of the Superstrong Black Mother, there have sometimes been fathers (and Otherfathers) present, and they, too, have struggled to change in order to better care for the children in their families. The task of care is not the only possible ground project that constitutes a life, of course. It is not always the central ground project for all the family members I have written about—at least not during some periods of their lives. But analytically, this project is certainly as strong a candidate as any other as a "moral engine" of everyday life, especially in light of the necessary interdependence of humans upon one another. We humans simply would not exist individually or collectively without being, at times in our lives, a central ground project for significant others.

I have tried to be as explicit as possible about how my first person virtue ethics with its moral laboratories departs from alternative ethical imaginaries currently circulating in anthropology and related disciplines. The most important point of departure is an analytic insistence on first person moral selves. This has meant foregrounding an "I" not as an autonomous actor but in relationship to a prior intersubjective "we" and an "I" connected to significant others. Since intersubjectivity precedes individual subjectivity, the first person plural is more fundamental than its singular counterpart. And yet, I have claimed, individual selves are indispensable conceptually. This perspective is most strongly supported by Anglo-American virtue ethics, with their "thick" version of the moral self. It is in light of this claim that a first person virtue ethics parts company most decisively with discursive moral frameworks.

The second point of departure, locating moral agency (including deliberate ethical reflection on norms) within the moral ordinary, has involved privileging the *singular event,* directing my gaze to the particularities of experience. I have tried to problematize the view that everyday life primarily involves unreflective and nondeliberative norm-following. Of course, people do not deliberate about everything all of the time. Any adequate virtue ethics that takes moral experience seriously must recognize the importance of its habitual and nondeliberative aspects. This is why Murdoch's notion of "moral re-orientation" (or what I have called "narrative re-envisioning"), with its experiential and embodied dimensions, offers a better picture of moral becoming than philosophy's dominant ideas of moral willing and free choice that overstate the conscious deliberative moment. However, if moral life concerns ongoing attempts to realize ground projects, if we take the *temporality* of morality seriously, in other words, then we can see that small moments and routine activities that, at first glance, appear repetitious, prereflective, or inconsequential come to take on depth as episodes in unfolding narratives of moral striving and as part of conscious commitments to realize particular versions of the good life.

A third point of departure concerns the importance of potentiality or hope in everyday life. Anthropology's methods of carrying out fieldwork and its careful attention to the intricacies of everyday life mean that it is poised to do an unmasking of the ordinary not merely as a darker and less promising place than we had thought but also as a more transcendent place. Training our scholarly gaze upon reality as a space of possibility and hope is equally important as cultivating skeptical insight and theories. Anthropologists are situated to explore possibility *concretely* through studies of how people, on the ground and in the midst of living their lives try to discern it. This is to be assessed only by taking a first person perspective on the possibilities for transformation and change seriously. No third person consideration of structural conditions of possibility, however useful, can supersede or foreclose this close investigation of the possible. Transformations directed to realizing a good life, especially for the disenfranchised, are more likely to emerge from the ground up and not the top down. This demands the need for small histories, histories of the nearly invisible, bringing to light efforts that would otherwise be unnoticeable.

I have taken the perspective of actors themselves as a serious analytic starting point. But by adopting a first person perspective, I do not mean that analysis should end with people's self-declarations. The point of ethnographic work is not to offer some kind of imitation of authentic indigenous meaning, some mirror of the "native's point of view," as we once used to say. Even if this were possible (and of course it is not), the point of ethnography is not to textually mirror what others have said and done. Rather, what matters is unmasking the *profoundness* that lies beneath the surface of the ordinary. It concerns making visible the actions, commitments, and struggles of people in ways that are often disguised because, from an inside or indigenous perspective, these are just everyday, just part of how life is, of what one does. Discovering and illuminating the drama of ordinary life is one of anthropology's most important unmasking tasks.

This has also involved disclosing the tragic potential of transformative projects. The ordinariness that comes with a life of chronic suffering, especially when combined with poverty and racism, the sheer day-to-dayness of it, can mean that participants themselves do not notice or respect their own hard work. They may not sufficiently acknowledge the moral double binds that their situations have put them in. They blame themselves or are blamed by others because the daunting intransigence of their problems is somehow hidden. Uncovering the enormity of the task of realizing moral dreams, or even the tragedy of moral incommensurabilites, not only helps reveal where key obstacles to transformation lie. It also speaks to the deep demoralization that very often occurs when people cannot find any enduring paths toward changing their personal, familial, and communal lives.

THE MORAL ORDINARY REVOLUTIONIZED

Throughout this book I have suggested what a narrative—and revolutionized—first person virtue ethics might look like, one that foregrounds projects of struggle for a "good life" that is especially directed to care of the other, and one that takes our human singularity and the dialogical nature of our intersubjective life as primary. I have drawn upon the features that have generally characterized neo-Aristotelian virtue ethics.

But it has been essential to "revolutionize" Aristotle in ways that take into consideration features of social life that were certainly of concern in ancient Athens but have been most energetically articulated by the past hundred and fifty years of critical social theory. These social features include the insidious role of power and inequality that pervades human relations, the way that power and knowledge are bound up together, and the necessity for reflection and critique upon the very categories and norms that guide moral action.

A focus on events permits us to see how everyday practice can have the potential not to be a mere repetition or reproduction of a habitus but also a space of dramatic moments of experimentation and revolution. Although I have distanced myself from a simple resistance-subjection dichotomy, I use the term *revolution* quite literally here in one important sense. The transformative work I have examined is not confined to projects of self-development; it also demands that the world be changed. That world may be centered primarily in the sphere of the family, but it almost inevitably leads to a gradual recognition that the care of intimate others demands negotiation, problematization, and sometimes direct confrontation with institutions and their modes of expert care or with modes of everyday community life.

In stressing the experimental uncertainty of moral life, I have insisted that moral becoming does not occur in a world of already realized ends. Ernst Bloch, a philosopher who has written brilliantly about hope, argues that *only* when the past can be seen in its contingency (from the perspective of what might have been otherwise) can it provide a ground for action directed to *change* rather than repetition of the past. He calls this imaginative access to the real the "principle of hope." This principle of hope reveals the "essence" of something that "is not-yet-being" (Bloch 1988:343). From this stance, we discover: "The inheritance that is to be claimed from the past . . . is not a legacy of fixed tradition, but of undischarged hope-content" (Bloch 1988:xxvii). The "real," Bloch proclaims, is process, a process that is—most importantly—*unfinished* as it mediates among present, unfinished past, and, above all, possible futures (1988:196).

In offering scenes of everyday life as moral laboratories and not just moral prisons or artisanal guilds, I have tried to suggest that it is essential to attend to an indigenous hermeneutics of hope, experiment, and creativity. Thus I have offered brief glimpses into everyday spaces that become "moral laboratories" in which people consider, and reconsider, the moral good. And yet, these moments I have sketched do not necessarily document transformative successes. Rather they are living experiments in which the outcomes are still very much in suspense and in which the odds are often stacked against every hope. What they reveal, in fact, is what Aristotle took to be so essential to practice—its character as a process. To speak of these experiments in a more political way, they show us processes in which people sometimes try to change their lives, to make history, not because they have some heroic capacity for transcendence but because they do not see any other chance for themselves, because it is too tragic not to try, no matter the odds. Part of the tragedy of projects of moral and political transformation is their ephemeral nature, the difficulty of getting any solid purchase on a trajectory of change that can have a lasting effect.

Das (2007) speaks of the work of those living in poverty and violence as a determined "descent into the ordinary." Although the ordinary is often distinguished from the extraordinary and the dramatic, she emphasizes how the ordinary sometimes becomes, in fact, something wondrous, an essential source of hope, what she calls a "temporality of second chances" (2007:101). Her argument resonates powerfully with my own, as she states emphatically, it is not enough to see how "the experience of becoming a subject is linked . . . to the experience of subjugation." Rather, one must also see how subjects remake their lives in the face even of violent domination. As Das and Kleinman put it, "While everyday life is fraught with the potential of danger . . . it is in the institutions of everyday life itself that we find the making of hope" (2000:10). This "descent into the ordinary" speaks to a type of transcendence that does not leave ordinary life behind but tries to move toward it, to inhabit it, to cultivate it. In Arendt's "beginnings," Das's "second chances," and my "narrative experiments" and "moral laboratories," we can hear an insistence upon the ordinary as a space in which something new can be created, however fragile and unpredictable its consequences.

I return one last time to the families I have introduced to convey this ethnographically.

HISTORY WITH A SMALL *h*: UNFINISHED EXPERIMENTS

Tanya

Tanya, the "soccer mom" introduced in the first chapter, continues to be a political activist in her community. Her transformation into this activist role continues, especially with the Los Angeles school system. Much of it has centered on battles with the schools her son has attended. She has been in a persistent battle with the principal and other teachers of regular education classes. She has banded together with fellow parents of children with special needs. As her frustration and skepticism grows, so does the scope of her challenge. After years of unsuccessful attempts to have children with disabilities included in regular education activities at the wealthy white school, she moved her son back into the local and much poorer school in her Inglewood neighborhood. Although initially she thought wealthy white parents would make more effective political allies than poor African American ones, she has changed her mind. "I'm making more headway here, even though there's no funds, no resources." She shakes her head in bewildered surprise.

Dotty and Betsy

Betsy is eighteen at the time of this writing. She never had a bone marrow transplant. As Dotty continued to explore this option and talked it over with Dr. Carter, she finally concluded that perhaps she should give this hope up. Perhaps this experimental procedure was indeed too risky, not only because of her daughter's many medical frailties but because an unrelated donor transplant had the potential for too many dangerous side effects. Perhaps in the future, when the technology has been developed further, there could be another chance for this, she has concluded. Looking back, she has worried that she was too willing to take a chance on such an experimental procedure. "Maybe I was just hoping for some kind of miracle," she has commented.

Meanwhile, as Betsy has gotten older, new problems have become paramount. As a teenager, she has been going through a rebellious phase where she doesn't want to take her medications as she should. Her iron levels have sometimes gotten dangerously high as a result. Equally worrisome, the chronic pain she has experienced over the years has troubled the clinicians and Dotty herself. Could it be that her daughter is becoming dependent upon the highly addictive medications that she has used all these years to control her pain? Or could her body be developing a resistance to the pain medications after all these years? "This can't just be my fight anymore," Dotty has said. "Betsy is getting older. This is her body. She has got to fight for her own health now. I can't just do it for her."

In coming to grips with this realization, Dotty faces a new moral dilemma. What does it mean to be a good mother who continues to be protective but, at the same time, somehow lets her child go? One of the reasons Dotty was so committed to pursuing the experimental bone marrow operation when Betsy was younger was because she feared this time when she would not have the same control over her daughter, when her daughter would have the choice to refuse care or refuse to take her medications as prescribed, or where none of the treatments that had worked in the past were effective any longer. There is also the possibility of becoming seriously addicted to the drugs. She dreaded these possibilities when her daughter was younger, and now some of her worst fears may be coming true. Dotty is also tired. She says she is just too tired, bone tired. She wants a "life of her own" now. "I feel like Stella," she jokes. "I want my groove back." But she also doesn't know what that even means. What would it even mean to be a person who is not a Rambo Mother, fighting for her daughter's life every single day? Who would she be? Maybe she should seriously consider dating, she muses.

In Greek tragedies, the main characters usually die. If they have faced moral incommensurabilities, these remain for the audience to ponder, but the protagonists leave the stage. In real life, however, people may live on. How has Dotty faced the morally incommensurable situation she was caught in when her daughter was younger? She has changed the stage. As with Tanya, fighting for better care for her daughter has meant moving into an increasingly politicized position. Over the years, Dotty has been called upon to be a speaker at various sickle cell conferences, representing the family's perspective. She is becoming more active in this organization. "Now that Betsy is older I'm ready to get involved in a bigger way, fight for people with sickle cell." She has always been conscious of the race connection to this illness, and the lack of funding for experimental drugs and procedures that she recognizes is linked to its identity as a "black disease." She has been taking the "Rambo" character she has cultivated to a larger venue, fighting not simply for her own daughter's care but for the whole group of people who suffer not only from this disease but from a host of serious chronic illnesses like her daughter's.

> I'm not interested in running a sickle cell support group. I've tried that. That doesn't work. I'm not interested in that. I think my interest is a lot broader than that. I'm interested in making a significant change. . . . I'm not interested in running a group. I want to see changes in the way kids are being treated in the hospital, in the way the parents are being treated. I want them to be more empowered. I want them to be more responsible for their kids, for themselves. And I want them to start producing adults that can be contribut-

ing members of society. That's what I want. I don't want kids who think they are going to be dead by the time they are twenty because they can't get good care. I don't want that.

Though Tanya speaks of growing tired and disillusioned, she also sees her increasingly political efforts as one possible avenue to provide better care for her son as well as other children. But Dotty is not in the same position. She has taken a more political role not because it is an improvement over a more intimate familial maternal one but because now that her daughter has gotten as old as she has, she no longer has the same power to control what happens to her. Dotty's political work, in other words, is not simply a political story but also a story about futility and finding a way to deal with her own pain at her daughter's uncertain future. She says that in deciding to become a political activist for the sickle cell community and potentially for an even broader one, she hopes that she can alleviate some of her own pain.

> And as a result of doing that I think I will be able to help myself alleviate some of my own issues, pain, whatever. And that's what I plan to do. I'll do it. I'll do it one way or another.

She sees her primary motivator as fear—fear is what propels her to action because the alternative is too terrible to live with. The longer she has had experience with sickle cell, the more it has made her afraid. This is what has moved her toward political activism.

> The greatest motivator in life is fear. Anybody who is afraid of something will be motivated to do something. Because if you don't do something you will sit there and you will just, it will just smother you. I am afraid, I am deathly afraid of sickle cell. I respect it. Initially, I thought I could control it, but I can't. So I respect it and I recognize it for what it is. It's no friend of mine, but it is a very good motivator. It's a very, very good motivator. And I am scared to death. And that, that's what keeps me going. That's what keeps me going.

Andrew and Darlene

It will come as no surprise that Arlene, the baby in the neonatal intensive care unit who had so many surgeries, died when she was eighteen months old. The doctors had never expected her to live as long as she did but, as Andrew and Darlene continued to say, this was because of their insufficient faith in God's hand. When she died they were determined to bury her properly, so that she could have a gravesite. Though they were too poor to pay for this, in the days after her death they quickly raised money by organizing a hot dog sale in the neighborhood. They not only raised enough money to bury, her but they were even able to buy a plaque with her name on it that they could put up in the halls of the hospital. Everyone at the hospital was surprised, they told us. "They didn't think we could afford something like that!" For months after she died, Andrew continued to drive to the hospital almost daily. "I don't know why," he told us. "It just seems like that became my life. The car just drives itself."

Arlene's death was only one of many disasters that befell them. Andrew went to prison for three months for a traffic offense. (This happened under California's "three strike" rule.) He might have been able to pay a large fine to get out of the sentence but they couldn't afford to. Since the family had no money, he did the time. Then there was the armed robbery by some neighborhood boys, and they and their children were held up at gunpoint at home, an incident I recounted in an earlier chapter. A few months after they moved out of the South Central area that had always been their home, Darlene had a stroke. Andrew had already had one stroke (he had diabetes) but he had recovered. Darlene, who also had diabetes and high blood pressure, suffered a severe stroke that left her substantially paralyzed. "I'll just take care of her the way we did Arlene," Andrew told us five years ago. That was the last time we heard from them. We have continued to send invitations to our collective narrative groups and "family reunions" with the research team, but there has been no response. Sometimes our cards are returned to us marked "Addressee unknown."

Delores's Family: Willy, Sasha, Marcy, Ralph

This is one of the most complicated stories of all. Willy is now thirteen years old. He is small for his age and the scars on his face are still prominent. He will need more surgeries in the future to minimize scarring. His mother is considering when there would be a good time to do this. But this medical story is a very small part of the picture of this extended family's life, a minor tragedy in what has been an apparently relentless downfall that has torn this family apart again and again. Here are a few of the key incidents.

In November 2006, Willy's father was shot and killed in front of a cousin's house while Willy was inside. He and Sasha had been engaged to be married the following spring. In January 2007, when Delores died, the family fractured in a way that continued for another two years. In April 2007 there was an arrest of several members of the family for drug dealing, including Sasha. She went to prison where she served nearly a year's term and then spent three months in a halfway house. She was still in prison in January 2008 when Leroy was murdered. When he was shot, Willy had come outside with him and was standing just a few feet away. I have already mentioned his remarkable speech at Leroy's funeral that suggested a powerful presence that could allow him to hold his own, even with his grandmother dead and his mother in prison.

In the midst of this onslaught of misery, Marcy has continued to change. She still has the toughness that she'd always had, but even her voice has changed. She has sounded more and more like her mother. She has commented that others have remarked about this. "Yes, there's nobody left now that my mother is gone. It's up to me to take her place. I've got to be her now," she has said.

At the time of this writing, Sasha has recently married. By all accounts, Willy is thriving. Sasha holds out great hope for him. Ralph, who was seriously depressed for a long time after Leroy's death, has had a second child with his longtime girlfriend, and they have moved into their own place. After Leroy's death, he made some attempts to work with a local police-run unit trying to control neighborhood violence, but that did not work out for him for long. Marcy says he is doing better now emotionally but he has not been easy for me to get in touch with, so I do not know how things really are.

Andrena

> There is a loneliness that can be rocked. Arms crossed, knees drawn up; holding, holding on, this motion, unlike a ship's, smooths and contains the rocker. It's an inside kind—wrapped tight like skin. Then there is a loneliness that roams. No rocking can hold it down. It is alive, on its own. A dry and spreading thing that makes the sound of one's own feet going seem to come from a far-off place. —Toni Morrison, Beloved (1987: 521–522)

I conclude with Andrena, whose efforts of moral transformation were not as politicized as some of the other parents. Belinda, of course, has died. Andrena has as well. In the months and years after Belinda's death Andrena struggled to make a new life for herself. She vowed never to return to her old job as a receptionist in a car dealership. That life was over. She did part-time work caring for the children of two well–to–do families, chauffeuring them to various after-school events and, in general, mothering them in the absence of their very busy professional parents. She had to move from the apartment where she had lived since Belinda's sickness, because once her daughter died, she no longer received benefits that allowed her to pay the rent. Because Section 8 housing (government-subsidized housing) has become increasingly defunded in Los Angeles during recent years, she decided to move to a town about an hour's drive from central LA where she was born and raised, and where her older daughter and other members of her family still lived. There she managed to find a decent apartment that she could afford.

What she defined as her main job didn't pay her anything at all. She was a relentless volunteer for the hospital where her child was treated, working with a family cancer group who raised money for the hospital and to support cancer treatment. She became a central figure in this advocacy group, and she hoped that they would consider bringing her on as a paid liaison to work with other families. They had one funded position, but instead the family advocacy group hired another mother, a wealthy white woman whose child had also recently died. Andrena spoke to me several times about her disappointment. She felt there was something unfair about this decision; she put in more hours than anyone and worked with more families (crossing race and ethnic lines) providing support and advice. Indeed, whenever I visited her, there were always families whose children were in the hospital on the phone with her. Although she was careful not to couch her disappointment in openly racial terms, she clearly wondered whether or not this was in part a racial decision. "You know there aren't so many blacks who go to this hospital anymore," she told me. "The area's changed too. Now it's much more Hispanic." She left unspoken, though hinted at, the growing tension that has arisen between Latinos and blacks in South Central Los Angeles in the past decades as Latinos have gradually moved into neighborhoods that were once African American strongholds.

Andrena's economic situation grew much worse when the primary family who had been paying her to care for their children suddenly moved to Singapore. She was searching for other families who might hire her, but the bills were piling up. Early one morning in November 2003, three weeks after I had been to her fiftieth birthday party, I got a call from her twenty-eight-year-old daughter. "My mom's died," her daughter told me. "We just found her last night. The funeral will be this Friday." I simply couldn't believe it. "What?" I asked. "How can this be? How can she be dead? I just saw her." "I know," her daughter replied.

But she said it quietly, I realized after I hung up. She didn't even sound very surprised. I never explicitly asked just how Andrena had died, and she didn't volunteer any information. I remembered uneasily that when I saw Andrena at her birthday party, although she was beautifully dressed and poised, she had seemed especially tense. I had taken along the man I had recently started dating to meet her. (The man who is now my husband.) When I introduced him, she smiled with approval. She had seen me go through the difficult break-up of a long relationship and I could tell that she liked this new person in my life. "You'll be alright Cheryl," she said to me that night. I didn't think much about those words at the time, but after I got her daughter's call I wondered if she was saying good-bye. Her blood pressure had been very high, dangerously high, since Belinda's illness. She kept joking to me that she really needed to start dieting, but she couldn't seem to find the energy. Could she have had a sudden stroke? A heart attack? Or had she done something more deliberate?

Andrena's funeral was packed. Every seat was taken, and people stood in the back and around the seats of the church located in the heart of the South Central neighborhood where Andrena had grown up. There were Latino families, black families, and even a few white families as well. The speeches were charged not only with sadness and fondness but also with anger. There were funny and touching stories from childhood friends, family members, some of the parents Andrena had befriended at the hospital. There were a few frustrated and even bitter stories as well. One young woman in her early twenties, Andrena's niece, recounted a moment about a year earlier when she was in terrible emotional trouble. She was driving down the highway when suddenly she recognized the license plate of the car in front of her. It read "Belinda." She realized that this was Andrena's car—just the person who could help her out. She started honking her horn and Andrena, seeing her, motioned for her to pull over. They stopped by the side of the road. Andrena held her as she cried and then they went to have coffee and talk things over. At the funeral, this niece concluded her story with angry tears: "Why did she just have to help everyone else and not ask for help herself? Why didn't she lean on us? Why didn't she take better care of herself?" Several people nodded as she spoke.

I never found out exactly what happened to Andrena. Her daughter and I promised to talk later, after things had settled down, but we never did. I simply couldn't bear to call. When I finally tried, some months later, her daughter's phone had been disconnected. A few months after that I got her phone number from another parent in the study who knew the family. And yet, I have never tried to contact her. I know that she herself changed jobs. She had been working in a receptionist position, rather like the work Andrena once did. After Belinda died, Andrena talked her into training as a nurse's aide. She graduated from a program at her local community college, pleasing Andrena immensely. As far as I know, she still works in the same hospital where her sister got care, the hospital where Andrena spent so much time in the last six years of her life. I haven't run into her there, but I could find Andrena's daughter pretty easily if I wanted to. Perhaps someday I will.

PHILOSOPHICAL ANTHROPOLOGY: THE ANTHROPOLOGICAL CONTRIBUTION

This book represents an extensive conversation with some of the people I have come to know but also with philosophy—virtue ethics and phenomenology in particular. In the process of bringing this philosophical conversation into dialogue with ethnographic material and with anthropological scholarship, I haven't tried to use my material as case examples for ready-made philosophical theory. Instead, I have drawn upon philosophical as well as anthropological voices to think with, amending them as I have considered the narrative form of moral experience, the experimental features of ordinary life and the revolutionary potential of even authoritative discourses and imaginaries. I introduced the term "philosophical anthropology" in the first chapter, referencing Lear's (2006) description of it as an exploration of moral possibility. What do we learn about moral possibility from our own ethnographic travels? How might it further a dialogue between philosophy and anthropology? One answer concerns the stubborn ambiguity that life "on the ground," as we say, reveals and that anthropology can document so meticulously. Ambiguously, from the shadows of uncertain lives, it may shine attention on the close companionship between moral tragedy and moral possibility.

I offer a final example to illustrate, returning to Andrena's death. For a long time I was unwilling to write about how her life ended. She was the central character in my previous book, *The Paradox of Hope*. In the book's epilogue, I purposely refrained from mentioning her death or the puzzling circumstances surrounding it. At the time the *Hope* book came out, in 2010, she had been dead for six years. It was ambiguity, moral ambiguity, that stopped me. How could I speak of it without the "Blue

Balloons" chapter, which I had already determined would be part of a subsequent book on morality? What I didn't want was for people to categorize her death as a mere unhappy ending, a sympathetic dismissal. Something more was at stake. It also said something about possibility and the good life, and in several ways.

Most obviously, it exemplifies one kind of moral tragedy, in the ancient sense and as discussed by Nussbaum (1986, 2009). Moral tragedy, it will be remembered, classically concerned not merely unhappy endings but situations in which people act against their own evaluations of the good. If we accept Nussbaum's interpretation of how moral tragedy functioned for Athenians, these plays were not merely, or even primarily, existential meditations on human finitude and the role of fate in our lives. Rather—or additionally—they provided occasions to revisit the haunting question of whether something could have been done—by humans—to change the circumstances faced by the doomed heroes in the play. The tragedies provided resources for societal level cultural critique and questions about social justice. Andrena's suicide, if it was that, has just such tragic features. It manifestly exposes how cruelly consequential the social injustices that attended her situation can be. Having a child with a rare and ultimately fatal cancer might be considered a matter of bad luck well beyond human control (at least for now) but the economic straits she found herself in, her inability to find a financial way to support herself in the aftermath of Belinda's death or to find work worthy of her newfound skills and wisdom—this, surely, is in the realm of things that can humanly be changed. In this sense, her death invites moral outrage. How is it that someone from such a wealthy country should be required to survive the death of her daughter with so few financial resources, so little societal support?

And yet, something else also rings true here, suggesting that we continue to pay close attention to the first person features of Andrena's situation, the particulars that shaped the destiny that became hers. Although suicide was the one moral act Andrena had struggled most strenuously to avoid, the single choice she found most morally repugnant, her death signaled more than surrender. Or so it has gradually seemed to me. There was a layer of complexity about it that resisted any clear-cut understanding, even in her own moral terms. There was, after all, the packed church at her funeral, standing room only, filled not only with family and old friends but those Andrena had befriended at the hospital. She had lived four long, hard years after her daughter's death, and the overflowing church was a testimony to her efforts. Once, years later, I remarked plaintively to another parent who had known Andrena as long as I had: "Oh, I still miss her." The mother retorted with uncharacteristic sharpness, "She's with her baby and her mother now." It was clear that I had spoken out of turn. I thought for a long time about what this mother was trying to tell me. Andrena, her rebuke implied, had lived the best "good life" available. She had struggled. She had straggled. She had helped many people along the way. Enough was enough. As I thought this through, I wondered if Andrena had been working out a way to die as a moral possibility not available to her at her daughter's passing. If "care of the intimate other" was Andrena's ground project (as it surely was), when she lost Belinda, hadn't she extended this community of others to include so many of us sitting in that crowded church? Hadn't her years of struggle and straggle created an expanding "we" or some transformed individuals? Certainly I was one of them, for I had learned a lot from her about staying close to someone through death, as she had done with Belinda. In all this "suffering for," to remember Throop's Yapese, perhaps Andrena had managed to craft a new moral possibility for herself. We, the living who sat side by side on the pews, were witnesses of a sort. Perhaps her continued membership with the living meant that, even by her own strict evaluative standards, leaving could finally emerge as a moral best good.

These speculations about Andrena are surely not definitive, but they do raise an important question about moral possibility as it can be explored through anthropology. Andrena's life and the other lives I have written about offer provocations for an anthropology of morality that keeps suffering and the moral good in very intimate contact. It is no minor matter that we humans are immersed in lives where things are morally at stake in ways that demand ethical evaluation, creativity and the cultivation of character. It is a very good thing that some recent work in the anthropology of morality challenges an overly deterministic or victim-focused account of people's lives. However, my own fieldwork suggests to me that these moral dimensions, even at their most creative, cannot easily be extricated from the suffering that so often engenders reflection and experiment. These two figures, what Robbins (2013) has called the "suffering subject" and the "morally striving subject" (as reflective moral evaluator or experimenter), are more than close neighbors. Together they portray something indissoluble. It might even be called the human condition.

Notes

1. Minkler and Roe 1993; Okazawa-Rey 1994; Poindexter and Linsk 1999.

2. A more detailed discussion of this problematization is taken up in chapter 5.

3. Sharp and Ipsa 2009.

4. Collins 2000:157.

5. Blackman 1999.

6. Beauboeuf-Lafontant 2007.

7. Beauboeuf-Lafontant 2007; Blackman 1999; Collins 2000; hooks 1992; Miles 2008; Sanders and Bradley 2005; Sharp and Ipsa 2009.

8. hooks 1992.

9. Beauboeuf-Lafontant 2007:32.

10. Zigon (2010) has usefully proposed the notion of a "moral assemblage," drawing upon the notion of cultural assemblages in the work of Ong and Collier (2008) in particular.

11. Robbins notes that it was rooted in a utopianist promise that, elsewhere, there might be cultures that knew how to live good lives that we (Westerners) could not imagine. He quotes Schneider on this point: "'One of the fundamental fantasies of anthropology is that somewhere there must be a life really worth living'" (1967:viii, in Robbins 2013: 456).

12. For example, in a fascinating study of the Ik, an infamously "cruel" people as depicted by Colin Turnbull, the Ik contend that their amoral and cruel acts only occur during historical periods of extreme starvation but ordinary morals and ideals are reinstated as soon as they once again have enough food to survive (Willerslev and Meinert, n.d.).

13. As Crowell puts it, "The fact that natural and social properties" can be used to describe us "is not sufficient to determine what it is for me to be a

human being. . . . Such properties are never merely brute determinations of who I am but are always in question" (Crowell 2010).

14. Perhaps no one in anthropology has taken up this issue so systematically and helpfully as the anthropologist Michael Jackson. See, especially, *Existential Anthropology* (2005).

15. This important phenomenological claim is often credited to Husserl, but Ricoeur traces it from Augustine and develops it in his own important work on time and narrative. For an anthropological treatment and development of this conception of lived time, see Mattingly 1998a, 2000, 2010a.

16. Arendt 1958; Baracchi 2008; MacIntyre 1981, 1988, 1990; Ricoeur 1978; Taylor 1985.

17. Baracchi 2008.

18. Although this is a common analogy in philosophical hermeneutics, it is taken up in more literary terms in Iser's remarkable book *The Act of Reading: A Theory of Aesthetic Response* (1980).

19. In a wonderfully illuminating essay on "historical experience" and narrativity as a response, see Wentzer's essay (2014).

20. Taylor builds upon Heidegger's discussion of the temporal structure of being—especially Heidegger's essential argument that we are most essentially beings who *become*—to make a strong case for narrative identity that is, at base, a moral identity. "From my sense of where I am relative to 'the good,' and among different possibilities, I project the direction of my life in relation to it. My life always has this degree of narrative understanding, that I understand my present action in the form of an 'and then': there was A (what I am), and then I do B (what I project to become)" (1989:47).

21. This feature of the self has been explored in the context of illness by a number of scholars, including Frank (1995, 2010), who has written with great explicitness about it.

22. A notable example is Fassin's extensive work. While not aligning himself with a specifically neo-Aristotelian approach, he tries to bring together the political and the ethical in subtle ways and situate anthropology within this and other moral frameworks adopted especially from philosophy. (For example see Fassin 2014.) Zigon provides another important example of this orientation to the ethical.

23. Faubion 2011; Zigon 2011.

24. See also Lambek 2010a, 2010b; Mattingly 1998b, 2012, 2013.

CHAPTER 2 FIRST PERSON VIRTUE ETHICS AND THE ANTHROPOLOGY OF MORALITY

1. As Robbins puts it, anthropology's focus on unfreedom" has placed it "in the vanguard of efforts to denaturalize the role notions of individual freedom play in various western ideologies" (2007:295).

2. For example, Parish (1994) has tried to make a place for moral choice by arguing that moral dictates have directive force but leave room for choice (see also Faubion 2001a). Lambek (2000, 2010a) draws upon Aristotle to oppose moral reasoning *(phronesis)* to unconscious moral acts or choices prompted by

strategic self-interest. See also Faubion 2001b, 2011; Mattingly 1998a; Laidlaw 2002, 2013; Lambek 2000, 2010b; Robbins 2004; Throop 2010b.

3. Laidlaw's more extended argument is as follows:

> Our discipline has not developed a body of theoretical reflection on the nature of ethics. I shall assume that this is a deficiency, and that it would therefore be an advance if it could be rectified. And my claim will be that in order to do so we shall need a way of describing the possibilities of human freedom: of describing, that is, how freedom is exercised in different social contexts and cultural traditions (2002:311).

4. Knight 2007; MacIntyre 1981, 1990; Mahmood 2005. Mahmood offers an especially useful summary of Aristotle's thought on Islamic religious practices. She offers an important clarification (2005:135–39) of Aristotle's notion of "habitus" as related to the cultivation of ethics, distinguishing it from the sense of unconscious predisposition as Bourdieu (1977) has developed the concept.

5. For example, Mahmood 2005; Robbins 2004; Throop 2010b; Zigon 2008, 2011.

6. Mattingly 2012.

7. For example; Annas 1995; Flynn 1997; Laidlaw 2013; Nehamas 1998; Paras 2006.

8. Brogan 2005; Hyland and Manousakis 2006.

9. Von Wright (1971) identified intentionalist explanation of action in terms of purpose and teleology (that is, first person agents whose behaviors needed to be understood as actions motivated by reasons and toward ends) as an Aristotelian tradition, one that stood as an important rival to various "causal" explanations being put forward in the social sciences that were trying to emulate the natural sciences. Aristotle's theory of practical reasoning offered a way to contest a monist theory of explanation borrowed from the natural sciences. Most important, rather than explaining action by subordinating particular acts under some form of general laws, the rationality of action could understood in terms of the actor's aspirations, intentions, and beliefs.

To give another example, such discussions and debates were also being developed around this time within philosophy of history, instigated especially by a famous challenge in which the philosopher of science Carl Hempel (1942) contended that historians who wrote "narrative histories" were insufficiently scientific because they lacked properly causal explanations based upon some kind of general laws—for example, underlying structural or psychological mechanisms that had predictive power. In other words, they were pre-explanatory and merely anecdotal. His challenge was met with a spirited defense of "narrative history" by some philosophers of history (for example, Dray 1957, *Laws and Explanations in History*, 1993, *Philosophy of History*). They countered that narrative histories were also explanatory but were based upon a different understanding of causation—one that linked actions to the intentional worlds of historical actors rather than to general laws that had predictive power in the way that physical laws, for example, could. And within the continental tradition of hermeneutic phenomenology, with Gadamer's work in particular, we also see how he calls upon Aristotle's concepts of practical reasoning and phronesis to contest the whole project of developing some standard form of "method" as a way to understand human action, experience and history.

10. Mattingly, Jensen, and Throop 2009; Anscombe 1957; Murdoch 1970.

11. MacIntyre (1981) argued that the family is the crucial moral sphere and advocates an "ethics of care" versus a more masculine version of ethics that has dominated traditional ideas of virtue.

12. Ochs 1988; Ochs and Capps 2001; Ochs and Kremer-Sadlik 2007. Keane notes that work in linguistic anthropology on child socialization has significant empirical evidence of how something like moral virtues are shaped through the cultivation of habits and emotions, and through such crucial speech genres as storytelling (Keane 2010).

13. As Laidlaw remarks, one can follow Foucault in defining freedom not as autonomous choice but as "something constructed out of the role given to choice in various cultures and in various domains within specific cultures (Laidlaw 2002:323).

14. Although [Foucault] maintained the distinction between technologies of power/domination and technologies of self, many scholars regard these as compatible. Foucault frequently spoke of the importance of considering their interdependence, providing numerous examples of "the point where the technologies of domination by individuals over one another have recourse to processes by which the individual acts upon himself and, conversely, the points where the technologies of the self are integrated into structures of coercion"(Foucault 1993:203) The distinction should be considered as a heuristic device and not the portrayal of two conflicting sets of interests (Powell and Biggs 2004). In fact, in choosing to highlight Foucault's influence, I foreground a particularly ambiguous figure. The late Foucault is maddening to pin down, as evidenced by the contradictory ways his last works have been read. While trying to avoid embroiling myself in some thankless hermeneutic enterprise of Foucault-reading, I just note that broadly speaking, there are two interpretative positions.

One position sees in his work threads or continuities in which his final works on subjectivity continue to outline problematics identified in his earliest works. From this interpretive perspective, one could claim that despite differences in emphasis and in subject matter (his earliest works being about truth, his middle period about power/governmentality, and his final works about subjectivity/care of the self), these three themes are connected and that Foucault himself saw them as interlacing: power/truth/subjectivity were mutually constitutive. A second reading is to see his final work on ethics as radically divorced from his earlier work and to treat his final work as in many ways compatible with neo-Aristotelian virtue ethics because Foucault explores ethical positions developed within Western antiquity.

15. See also Jay 2005.

16. The rejection of a first person position also encompasses a challenge to "commonsense" notions of truth and meaning. Foucault's initial genealogical work was heralded by anthropologists and philosophers as a means to get "beyond" humanist projects in which the dilemmas, self-interpretations, misunderstandings, and perplexities faced in everyday life were the material for moral

theorizing. So, Rabinow and Dreyfus declared, "Foucault is not interested in recovering man's unnoticed everyday self-interpretation. He would agree with Nietzsche and the hermeneutics of suspicion that such an interpretation is surely deluded about what is really going on" (Dreyfus and Rabinow 1983:xxiii).

This challenge is enormously provocative and destabilizing. Unlike, say, the hermeneutics of suspicion that characterized nineteenth-century critical theories (Marx and Freud most notably), in the Foucauldian challenge articulated here by Dreyfus and Rabinow, there is not a notion of a true or truer version of self-understanding that can be uncovered. In the spirit of Nietzsche, the search for meaning (as either a scholarly or an ordinary practical project) is construed as based upon mythical assumptions, a form of delusion. As Nietzsche famously asked (translated here by MacIntyre 1990), "What then is truth?"

> A mobile army of metaphors, metonymies, and anthropomorphisms, a sum, in short, of human relationships that, rhetorically and poetically intensified, ornamented and transformed, come to be thought of, after long usage by a people, as fixed, binding, and canonical. Truths are illusions that we have forgotten are illusions, worn-out metaphors now impotent to stir the senses, coins that have lost their faces and are considered now as metal rather than currency."

What the genealogist uncovers, then, is not truth or meaning in the hermeneutic sense but rather, how truths, subjectivities, notions of meaning are produced in any historical period through various social practices, that is, through forms of institutional governance, through the discourse of experts, through the training of bodies, through the organization of temporal and physical space, through a well-worn but "mobile army of metaphors."

Foucault's discussion of morality, even in his later work, is a continued reminder of the pervasive power of oppressive social structures. A great part of Foucault's genius lies in emphasizing what it is that people on the ground are *not* seeing and *not* knowing, and especially how they are blind to the institutional forces that constrain them. We can see this with startling clarity in an interview that Foucault did late in his career with two sympathetic and philosophically trained interviewers. Foucault sees our primary theoretical task as pointing out the dangers of contemporary society: "Everything is dangerous," he says. He argues for "a hyper- and pessimistic activism." Ethically speaking, the "choice we have to make every day is to determine which is the main danger" (Foucault in Dreyfus and Rabinow 1983:232).

17. But, for exceptions, see Das 2007, 2010; Lambek 2002b, 2003, 2008, 2010a, b; Mattingly 1998a, 1998b, 2010a, 2010b.

18. Many examples could be given here. Some notable ones include Willen (2010) and other work by Biehl and colleagues (Biehl and Moran-Thomas 2009).

19. As Lambek notes, "There is no great methodological danger in dissolving the ethical into the social once the social is couched as "(Aristotelian) activity, practice, and judgment rather than (Kantian/Durkheimian) rule or obligation" (2010b:28).

20. Lambek 2010a, 2010b; Mattingly 1998b, 2010b.

21. Jackson 1989, 1995, 1996, 2005, 2007.

22. Wikan 1990.

23. Kleinman 1999a, b; 2006.

24. Jackson 1989.

25. Csordas 1994, 2002; Desjarlais 1997; Throop 2003, 2010a, 2010b.

26. Desjarlais and Throop (2011) offer a concise review of this discussion and offer some key defenses of the phenomenological tradition and its first person orientation.

27. Notably Csordas 1994, 2002; Desjarlais 1992, 1996, 2003; Michael Jackson 1996, 2007.

CHAPTER 3 HOME EXPERIMENTS

1. For example, Faubion 2011; Laidlaw 2013; Mahmood 2005; Robbins 2004; Throop 2010b; Zigon 2008, 2011.

2. As Butler puts it:

> We start to give an account [of ourselves] only because we are interpellated as beings who are rendered accountable by a system of justice and punishment. . . . So I start to give an account . . . because someone has asked me to, and that someone has power delegated from an established system of justice. I have been addressed, even perhaps had an act attributed to me, and a certain threat of punishment backs up this interrogation. And so, in fearful response, I offer myself as an "I" and try to reconstruct my deeds, showing that the deed attributed to me was or was not, in fact, among them (2005:10–11).

3. Butler (1997, 2005) following Althusser has described this as "interpellation."

4. Agamben 1998; Butler 1997; Rose 1990; Zigon 2011.

5. This is because the deliberative aspects of the moral are often downplayed or disregarded. For example, when Mahmood reads Aristotle's ethics, she rightfully distinguishes "habitus" as Bourdieu takes up the term from habitus as given to us by Aristotle. She notes that Aristotle's original concept of habitus concerns the acquiring of moral excellence through repeated practice—through a kind of training that leaves its imprint on a person's character. This feature of moral becoming is what Bourdieu's account leaves out. However, when she argues that the result and even the aim of a moral practice is "making moral behavior a non-deliberative aspect of one's disposition" (2005:137), this parts company with much of the philosophical tradition of neo-Aristotelian virtue ethics that also continues to emphasize Aristotle's concern with complexities of *moral judgment*.

6. For example, Dave 2010; Faubion 2010, 2011; Zigon 2009. Thus, Faubion is concerned to distinguish between what he calls the "dynamic" aspects of self-creation and its "more homeostatic and reproductive aspects"—the "themitical" (2011:20). The dynamic scene "is one in which the typically subliminal themitical normativity of everyday routine is in suspension. . . . The scene of crisis is a scene of the unfamiliar or of disturbance, in which the experience of the disruption or of the failure of the reproduction of routine is also the impetus of thought and action" (2011:81–82). Zigon (2007, 2009) distinguishes the "moral," which he equates with an everyday, unconscious habitus provided by

the widely shared norms of one's society or communities, and the "ethical," which involves some "breakdown" in this habituated moral activity, thus presenting the actor with a situation that requires conscious deliberation. In everyday life, it is unquestionably the moral that predominates, Zigon argues. The ethical, by contrast, is much more rare; it is generated by the infrequent situation when "one actually has to stop and consider how to act or be morally appropriate" (2009:260).

7. One might reasonably ask for more detail about how this inaugural scene with its moral laboratories and journeys is narrative in a different way than, for example, the inaugural scene of a courtroom—which obviously also suggests the need for a narrative account of oneself and, therefore, both presupposes and creates a narrative version of a moral self. I continue to address this question in subsequent chapters.

8. I have developed this claim elsewhere in an extended way, offering a "narrative phenomenology" of action and experience (Mattingly 2010b).

9. He tells us that there is a "knowledge of oneself "that is "transcendental with respect to one's given subject position as defined by society" (2004: 154–55).

10. This complex portraiture is something I have tried to do in my own work, drawing especially upon virtue ethics and phenomenology (e.g., Mattingly 1998a, 1998b, 2006a, 2006b, 2009, 2010a, 2010b).

CHAPTER 4 LUCK, FRIENDSHIP, AND THE NARRATIVE SELF

1. I should mention that Arendt treats action, as I have described it here, in an ambiguous way. On the one hand, she valorizes the uncertainty of human affairs because of the frailties of action I have described and she has a great deal to say about natality. On the other hand, she tells us that action of this sort (praxis), where something new is begun, is rare (Arendt1958:178).

2. See also Throop 2010b.

3. It provides a training ground for inhabiting the subject position of the Superstrong Black Mother. For example, Sasha is explicit about how it has taught her strength, in "testing her faith," in "humbling her," and in forcing her to face the biggest challenge of her life. She contrasts her earlier self, a mother to be sure, but one who had not been so "tested":

> It was like a test of my faith. It humbled me a lot. Everything has always either been given to me or you know, always been provided. So this is something that I have to deal with myself. It was my test, you know? I guess it was supposed to happen.

CHAPTER 5 MORAL TRAGEDY

1. Dotty and Betsy have been written about using different pseudonyms (Noreen and Danielle respectively) in Mattingly 2010b:65–67.

2. Not all virtue ethics scholars agree with Nussbaum on this matter. Williams, for example, in *Moral Luck*, complains that Aristotle's thinking is plagued by "his unappetizing ideal of self-sufficiency" (1981:15). Nussbaum challenges this common reading of Aristotle in works such as *The Fragility of Goodness*

that were published after *Moral Luck*. But, as with Foucault, my purpose in this book is not to weigh in on the debate. Rather, I am following a line of argument (in this case Nussbaum's) that I find compelling and useful.

CHAPTER 6 THE FLIGHT OF THE BLUE BALLOONS

1. In a very compelling analysis of how stories work on us, Arthur Frank (2010) makes a strong case for the suspenseful self. This has been a central concern in my own work as well (Mattingly 1998b, 2000, 2010a, 2010b).

2. The proposal for a subjunctive or experimental self and, more broadly, attention to time and the narrative complexity of illness experience and clinical care has also been importantly explicated by Mary-Jo DelVecchio Good (1995) and Byron Good (1994). Jerome Bruner (1986, 1990) put the term "subjunctivity" into broad circulation in his seminal works on how people think with stories. Other scholars have also tried to complicate an overly coherent and linear depiction of the self by suggesting that there are multiple ways we experience and inhabit ourselves. Michael Lambek makes an intriguing claim along these lines. Although his emphasis is directed to the "public side of personhood rather than the interior and reflective life of the self or subject," he proposes that there are two "universal and intrinsic dimensions of the person" that have moral import. One is precisely the linear, cumulative self. But there is another kind of self (or person) possible that involves a kind of play on "impersonation" of societally offered personae that allow for the production of "discontinuous" and "non-unitary" persons (2013:838).

CHAPTER 7 RIVAL MORAL TRADITIONS AND THE MIRACLE BABY

1. There is a prodigious literature that documents this. See also Jordan 1978, 1989, 1997; Martin 1987. One response to this problematic biomedical aesthetic has involved the call to humanize medicine by paying much more explicit attention to its metaphors and narratives and by training clinicians to become more sensitive and self-aware of how they draw on these in their work. In fact, training in "narrative competence" has become one approach to help clinicians recognize the narrative features of their patient's experience and of their own practices. There are many contributing voices, but Rita Charon has been a pioneer here. (See Charon 2008; Charon and Montello 2002).

2. Bridges 2011; Fraser 1998.

3. Davis-Floyd and St. John 1998; Martin 1994; Weiss 1997, Frank 1995, Cassel 1991

4. Mattingly 2010b:68.

5. Contemporary science studies, and especially studies concerning the technoscience of biomedicine, have made it a point to unearth the figural behind the factual in how the body is conceived (Franklin and Lock 2003; Martin 1994; J. Taylor 2005). One might even consider, as some anthropologists have suggested, that it makes sense to "collapse magic, science and religion together as 'overlapping projects of world-making'" (Wiener 2003, 2004). And, I would

add, to recognize that none of these projects of world-making can do without figural grounding.

6. Hebert et al. 2001; Mansfield et al. 2002.

7. Abrums 2000, 2004; Bowen-Reid and Harrell 2002; Frazier 1974 [1963]; Grant 1989; Hine and Thompson 1998; hooks 1995; Richardson 1980). Not only do African Americans report substantially higher church affiliation (about 75 to 80 percent), as compared to white Americans (about 60 to 70 percent); their level of active involvement in church activities is markedly higher.

8. Chatters et al. 2002:66.

9. Ibid.

10. "Jesus is an ever-present friend who helps the faithful deal with everyday hardships, and gives them strength in their quest for freedom from oppressive traditions" (Abrums 2004:190).

11. Farran et al. 2003; Polzer and Miles 2005; Wilson and Miles 2001.

12. Grant 1989; Matthews, Lannin, and Mitchell 1994; for example, Hines and Boyd-Franklin 1996; Levin and Taylor 1997; Levin, Taylor, and Chatters 1994; Mansfield, Mitchell, and King 2002.

13. Navaie-Waliser et al. 2001; Nightingale 2003; Polzer and Miles 2005; Potts 1996; Sistler and Washington 1999; Wilson and Miles 2001.

14. Perhaps something else is also at work that explains the remarkable, ontological contrast between virtue ethics traditions and dominant modern understandings of scientific knowledge, expertise, and ethics. Perhaps what we call "Western modernity" and its beliefs about knowledge (an era "after virtue" as MacIntyre puts it; a "secular age" in Taylor's words) represents something very culturally unusual in the world's history and we can expect to find it in sharp contrast to religious traditions of any kind.

15. Of all places where a blues hope has been fostered, it is in the black church: "The black church tradition has made ritual art and communal bonds out of black invisibility and namelessness" (West in Gates and West 1996:102).

16. hooks puts it this way, speaking of her own religious background:
Liberatory religious traditions affirmed identification with the poor. Taught to believe that poverty could be the breeding ground of moral integrity, of a recognition of the significance of communion, of sharing resources with others in the black church.... That solidarity was meant to be expressed not simply through charity, the sharing of privilege, but in the assertion of one's power to change the world so that the poor would have their needs met, would have access to resources, would have justice and beauty in their lives" (1994:167–68).

17. Cited by West in West and Gates 1996:53.

18. Carolyn Rouse, who worked for several years as a researcher in this study, has also written movingly about this case and the use of this metaphor in a 2004 article.

CHAPTER 8 DUELING CONFESSIONS

1. Oliver defines "the streets" as "the network of public and semipublic social settings (e.g., street corners, vacant lots, bars, clubs, after-hours joints, convenience stores, drug houses, pool rooms, parks and public recreational

places, etc.) in which primarily lower and working-class Black males tend to congregate (2006:919).

2. Hannerz 1969, Oliver 2006, Franklin et al. 1999, White and Cones 1999.

3. Roberts 1998.

4. Ibid., 148.

5. "Black male unemployment on average is 2 times greater than the unemployment rate among White males. In addition, Black males earn 62 cents for every dollar earned by White males. Also, as a result of the decline of low-skill, high-wage heavy industrial jobs and the expansion of low-wage service jobs and high-wage, high-skill information and technology jobs, Black males have born the brunt of the loss of low-skill, high-wage manufacturing jobs" (Oliver 2006:918–19).

6. Banks 2006.

7. Berry and Looney 1996.

8. Huff 2008; Hughes and Short 2005; Papachristos 2009.

9. This centrality of the church in the moral imaginary of African Americans also holds for black ex-slave communities throughout what Gilroy (1993) has called the "black Atlantic." Many scholars have argued that the centrality of spirituality in African American life is partly an inheritance from West Africa. "Influenced by their African heritage as well as by racism and the historic power relations between privileged and oppressed racial groups in the United States, African Americans believe that the most vital aspect of being is spirituality . . . spirituality is intertwined in all aspects of life" (Polzer and Miles 2005: 234; See also Stewart 1997; Mbiti 1969; Conner and Eller 2004: 625).

10. Harmon 2006.

11. There is a "long tradition of faith-based initiatives and work in black communities [that] has been concerned with the health and well-being of individuals and families" (Taylor et al. 2000:73). As Blank et al. point out: "The Black church has served a dominant role as an informal social service provider throughout its history . . . Services provided include substance abuse assistance as well as health screenings, education, and support" (2002:1668). (Rogers-Dulan and Blackher 1995; Chatters et al. 2002).

12. "Black churches can offer healing responses to problems that are occasioned primarily by the oppressive social infrastructures of racism, sexism, and classism" (Eugene 1995:55–56).

13. (Markens et al. 2002:806). Black churches have also traditionally functioned as "support convoys" that families may turn to in helping them with care of ill or disabled family members (Taylor et al. 2000). In this way, healing takes on multiple meanings.

14. Abrums argues, "The black church has functioned as the center of power and social life within the African American community. It has offered a safe space for discourse, for resistance to objectification as 'the Other,' and for black women's activism.

15. hooks sees that, within this setting, African Americans 'have learned oppositional ways of thinking that enhance our capacity to survive and flourish'" (2004:190).

16. In part this fusion can be attributed to the way that African American churches grew up in urban centers. While Protestant churches required build-

ings for its congregations, the flooding of black migrants into what quickly became overcrowded urban neighborhoods meant that space was at a premium. As traditional religious denominations such as Baptists and Methodists became overcrowded, new "storefront" churches of small denominations grew up that could serve the needs of local worshippers. They tended to be less formal, more participatory and oriented to the local needs of the neighborhood (Chireau 2006:195).

17. Hicks 1994.

Bibliography

Abrahams, Roger D. 1974. "Black Talking on the Streets." In *Explorations in the Ethnography of Speaking*, edited by Richard Bauman and Joel Sherzer, 240–62. Cambridge: Cambridge University Press.

Abrums, Mary. 2000. "'Jesus Will Fix It after a While': Meanings and Health." *Social Science and Medicine* 50 (12):89–105.

———. 2004. "Faith and Feminism: How African American Women from a Storefront Church Resist Oppression in Healthcare." *Advances in Nursing Science* 27 (3):187–201.

Adamson, Christopher. 1998. "Tribute, Turf, and the American Street Gang: Patterns of Continuity and Change since 1820." *Theoretical Criminology* 2 (1):57–84.

Agamben, Giorgio. 1998. *Homo Sacer: Sovereign Power and Bare Life*. Translated by Daniel Heller-Roazen. Stanford, CA: Stanford University Press.

Alim, Tanya, Adriana Feder, Ruth Graves, Yanping Wang, James Weaver, Maren Westphal, Alonso, Angeliques et al. 2008. "Trauma, Resilience, and Recovery in a High-Risk African American Population." *American Journal of Psychiatry* 165 (12):1566–75.

Alonso, Alex. 2010. "Out of the Void—Street Gangs in Black Los Angeles." In *Black Los Angeles: American Dreams and Racial Realities*, edited by Darnell M. Hunt and Ana-Christina Ramon, 140–67. New York: New York University Press.

———. 2010, September 26. *LAPD Detains Grape Street Crip Member during the Middle of an Interview in Jordan Downs*. YouTube Interview, 3:22 minutes. http://www.youtube.com/watch?v = 9I41JbYDa9E

Annas, Julia. 1995. *The Morality of Happiness*. New York: Oxford University Press.

Anscombe, Elizabeth. 1957. *Intention*. Cambridge, MA: Harvard University Press.

———. 1958. "Modern Moral Philosophy." *Philosophy* 33 (124): 1–19.

Appadurai, Arjun, ed. 1986. *The Social Life of Things: Commodities in Cultural Perspective*. Cambridge: Cambridge University Press.

———. 1996. *Modernity at Large: Cultural Dimensions of Globalization*. Minneapolis: University of Minnesota Press.

Appiah, K. Anthony, and Amy Gutmann. 1996. *Color Conscious: The Political Morality of Race*. Princeton: Princeton University Press.

Arendt, Hannah. 1958. *The Human Condition*. Chicago: University of Chicago Press.

Aristotle. 1970. *Poetics*. Translated by G. Else. Ann Arbor: University of Michigan Press.

———. 1985. *Nicomachean Ethics*. Translated by Terence Irwin. Indianapolis: Hackett.

Banks, James. 2006. "Improving Race Relations in Schools: From Theory and Research to Practice." *Journal of Social Issues* 62 (3):607–14.

Baracchi, Claudia. 2006. "Contributions to the Coming-to-Be of Greek Beginning: Heidegger's Inceptive Thinking." In *Heidegger and the Greeks: Interpretive Essays*, edited by Drew A. Hyland and John Panteleimon Manoussakis, 23–42. Bloomington: Indiana University Press.

———. 2008. *Aristotle's Ethics as First Philosophy*. Cambridge: Cambridge University Press.

Barnes, Linda, Gregory Plotnikoff, Kenneth Fox, and Sara Pendleton. 2000. "Spirituality, Religion, and Pediatrics: Intersecting Worlds of Healing." *Pediatrics* 106 (4):899–908.

Barnes, Sandra L. 2005. "Black Church Culture and Community Action." *Social Forces* 84 (2):967–94.

Beardsley, Monroe C. 1962. "The Metaphorical Twist." *Philosophy and Phenomenological Research* 22: 293–307.

———. 1967. "Metaphor." In *Encyclopedia of Philosophy* (vol. 5), edited by P. Edwards. New York: Macmillan.

Beauboeuf-Lafontant, Tamara. 2007. "'You Have to Show Strength': An Exploration of Gender, Race, and Depression." *Gender and Society* 21(1): 28–51.

Becker, Gay. 1994. "Metaphors in Disrupted Lives: Infertility and Cultural Constructions of Continuity." *Medical Anthropology Quarterly* 8 (4):383–410.

Berry, Venise, and Harold Looney Jr. 1996. "Rap Music, Black Men, and the Police." In *Mediated Messages and African-American Culture: Contemporary Issues*, edited by Carmen Manning-Miller and Venise Berry, 263–77. Thousand Oaks, CA: Sage.

Bhabha, Homi. 1994. *The Location of Culture*. New York: Routledge.

Biehl, Joao. 2005. *Vita: Life in a Zone of Social Abandonment*. Berkeley: University of California Press.

Biehl, Joao, and Amy Moran-Thomas. 2009. "Symptom: Subjectivities, Social Ills, Technologies." *Annual Review of Anthropology* 38 (1):267.

Biehl, Joao, Byron J. Good, and Arthur Kleinman. 2007. "Introduction: Rethinking Subjectivity." In *Subjectivity: Ethnographic Investigations*. Vol. 7, edited by Joao Biehl, Byron J. Good, and Arthur Kleinman. Berkeley: University of California Press.

———, eds. 2007. *Subjectivity: Ethnographic Investigations*. Vol. 7. Berkeley: University of California Press.

Biehl, Joao, and Peter Locke. 2010. "Deleuze and the Anthropology of Becoming." *Current Anthropology* 51 (3):317–51.

Black, Max. 1962. *Models and Metaphors*. Ithaca: Cornell University Press.

———. 1979. "More about Metaphor." In *Metaphor and Thought*, edited by Andrew Ortony, 19–41. Cambridge: Cambridge University Press.

Blackman, Lorraine. 1999. "The UMOJA Principle in Action: African Americans Forging Twenty-First Century Families." *Journal of African American Studies* 4 (1):53–69.

Blakemore, Jerome, and Glenda Blakemore. 1998. "African American Street Gangs: A Quest for Identity." *Journal of Human Behavior in the Social Environment* 1 (2–3):203–23.

Blank, Michael, Marcus Mahmood, Jeanne Fox, and Thomas Guterbock. 2002. "Alternative Mental Health Services: The Role of the Black Church in the South." *American Journal of Public Health* 92 (10):1668–72.

Bloch, Ernst. 1986. *The Principle of Hope* (Vol. 1). Translated by Neville Plaice, Stephen Plaice, and Paul Knight. Cambridge, MA: MIT Press.

———. 1988. *The Principle of Hope* (Vol. 2). Translated by Neville Plaice, Stephen Plaice, and Paul Knight. Cambridge, MA: MIT Press.

Bourdieu, Pierre. 1977. *Outline of a Theory of Practice*. Translated by Richard Nice. Cambridge: Cambridge University Press.

Bowen-Reid, Terra, and Jules Harrell. 2002. "Racist Experiences and Health Outcomes: An Examination of Spirituality as a Buffer." *Journal of Black Psychology* 28 (1):18–36.

Boyd, Richard. 1979. "Metaphor and Theory Change: What is 'Metaphor' a Metaphor For?" In *Metaphor and Thought*, edited by Andrew Ortony, 481–532. Cambridge: Cambridge University Press.

Branch, William, Alexia Torke, and Robin Brown-Haithco. 2006. "The Importance of Spirituality in African-Americans' End-of-Life Experience." *Journal of General Internal Medicine* 21 (11):1203–5.

Bridges, Khiara. 2011. *Reproducing Race: An Ethnography of Pregnancy as a Site of Racialization*. Berkeley: University of California Press.

Brodsky, Anne. 1999. "'MAKING IT': The Components and Process of Resilience among Urban, African-American, Single Mothers." *American Journal of Orthopsychiatry* 69 (2):148–60.

Brody, Howard. 1987. *Stories of Sickness*. New Haven: Yale University Press.

Brogan, Walter. 2005. *Heidegger and Aristotle: The Twofoldness of Being*. Albany: State University of New York Press.

Browner, Carole, and H. Mabel Preloran. 2010. *Neurogenetic Diagnoses: The Power of Hope and the Limits of Today's Medicine (Genetics and Society)*. New York: Routledge.

Bruner, Edward. 1984. "Introduction: The Opening Up of Anthropology." In *Text, Play and Story*, edited by Edward Bruner, 1–16. Prospect, IL: Waveland.

———. 1986. "Ethnography as Narrative." In *The Anthropology of Experience,* edited by V.W. Turner and Edward Bruner, 139–57. Chicago: University of Illinois Press.

Bruner, Jerome. 1986. *Actual Minds, Possible Worlds.* Cambridge, MA: Harvard University Press.

———. 1990. *Acts of Meaning.* Cambridge, MA: Harvard University Press.

Burke, Kenneth. 1945. *A Grammar of Motives.* Berkeley: University of California Press.

Burton, Linda M. 1992. "Black Grandparents Rearing Children of Drug-Addicted Parents: Stressors, Outcomes, and Social Service Needs." *Gerontologist* 32 (6):744–51.

Burton, Richard D.E. 1997. *Afro-Creole: Power, Opposition, and Play in the Caribbean.* Ithaca, NY: Cornell University Press.

Butler, Judith. 1997. *Excitable Speech: A Politics of the Performative.* New York: Routledge.

———. 2005. *Giving an Account of Oneself.* New York: Fordham University Press.

Carr, David. 1991. *Time, Narrative, and History.* Bloomington: Indiana University Press.

Carrithers, Michael. 2005. "Anthropology as a Moral Science of Possibilities." *Current Anthropology* 46 (3):433–56.

Cavell, Stanley. 2004. *Cities of Words: Pedagogical Letters on a Register of the Moral Life.* Cambridge, MA: Harvard University Press.

———. 2005. *Philosophy the Day after Tomorrow.* Cambridge, MA: Harvard University Press.

Cassel, Joan. 1991. *Expected Miracles: Surgeons at Work.* Philadelphia: Temple University Press.

Champlin, Charles. 1985. "'Rambo's' Right-Wing Revisions." *Los Angeles Times,* July 14.

Charon, Rita. 2008. Honoring the Stories of Illness. New York: Oxford University Press.

Charon, Rita, and Martha Montello (Eds.). 2002. *Stories Matter: The Role of Narrative in Medical Ethics.* New York: Routledge.

Chatters, Linda, Robert Taylor, Karen Lincoln, and Tracy Shroepfer. 2002. "Patterns of Informal Support from Family and Church Members among African Americans." *Journal of Black Studies* 33 (1):66–85.

Chireau, Yvonne P. 2006. "Varieties of Spiritual Experience: Magic, Occultism, and Alternative Supernatural Traditions among African Americans in the Cities." In *The Black Urban Community: From Dusk Till Dawn,* edited by Gail Tate and Lewis Randolph, 1915–39. New York: Palgrave Macmillan.

Coles, Robert. 1988. *The Call of Stories: Teaching and Moral Imagination.* Cambridge, MA: Harvard University Press.

Collier, Stephen, and Andrew Lakoff. 2005. "On Regimes of Living." In *Global Assemblages: Technology, Politics, and Ethics as Anthropological Problems,* edited by Stephen J. Collier and Aihwa Ong, 22–39. Malden, MA: Blackwell Publishing.

Collins, Patricia Hill. 1999. "The Meaning of Motherhood in Black Culture." In *The Black Family: Essays and Studies*, edited by Robert Staples, 157–66. Belmont, CA: Wadsworth.

———. 2000. *Black Feminist Thought: Knowledge, Consciousness, and the Politics of Empowerment*. New York: Routledge.

———. 2004. *Black Sexual Politics: African Americans, Gender, and the New Racism*. New York: Routledge.

———. 2006. *From Black Power to Hip Hop: Essays on Racism, Nationalism, and Feminism*. Philadelphia: Temple University Press.

Conner, Norma, and Lucille Eller. 2004. "Spiritual Perspectives, Needs and Nursing Interventions of Christian African-Americans." *Journal of Advanced Nursing* 46 (6):624–32.

Connolly, William. 1985. "Taylor, Foucault, and Otherness." *Political Theory* 13 (3):365–76.

Crapanzano, Vincent. 2004. *Imaginative Horizons: An Essay in Literary Philosophical Anthropology*. Chicago: University of Chicago Press.

Craven, Christa. 2005. "Claiming Respectable American Motherhood: Homebirth Mothers, Medical Officials, and the State." *Medical Anthropology Quarterly* 19 (2):194–215.

Criminal Justice Center. 2005. "Review of Homicide Crime Statistics, County Reports." State of California Department of Justice, Office of the Attorney General Website. http://oag.ca.gov/crime/cjsc/criminal-justice-profiles.

Crowell, Steven. 2010. "Existentialism." In *Stanford Encyclopedia of Philosophy*, edited by Edward N. Zalta. Stanford, CA: Metaphysics Research Lab, Center for the Study of Language and Information. http:plato.standord.edu/entries/existentialism.

Csordas, Thomas J. 1994. *The Sacred Self: A Cultural Phenomenology of Charismatic Healing*. Berkeley: University of California Press.

———. 2002. *Body/Meaning/Healing*. New York: Palgrave.

———. 2013. "Morality as a Cultural System?" *Current Anthropology* 54 (5):523–46.

Cureton, Steven R. 2009. "Something Wicked This Way Comes: A Historical Account of Black Gangsterism Offers Wisdom and Warning for African American Leadership." *Journal of Black Studies* 40 (2):347–61.

Dailey, Dawn E., Janice C. Humphreys, Sally H. Rankin, and Kathryn A. Lee. 2011. "An Exploration of Lifetime Trauma Exposure in Pregnant Low-Income African American Women." *Maternal and Child Health Journal* 15 (3):410–18.

Das, Veena. 1994. "Moral Orientations to Suffering: Legitimation, Power, and Healing." In *Health and Social Change in International Perspective*, edited by Lincoln Chen, Arthur Kleinman, and Norma Ware. Cambridge, MA: Harvard University Press.

———. 2007. *Life and Words: Violence and the Decent into the Ordinary*. Berkeley: University of California Press.

———. 2010. "Engaging the Life of the Other: Love and Everyday Life." In *Ordinary Ethics: Anthropology, Language, and Action*, edited by Michael Lambek, 376–99. New York: Fordham University Press.

Das, Veena, and Arthur Kleinman. 2000. "Introduction." In *Violence and Subjunctivity,* edited by Veena Das, Arthur Kleinman, Mamphela Ramphele, and Pamela Reynolds, 1–10. Berkeley: University of California Press.

Dave, Naisargi N. 2010. "Between Queer Ethics and Sexual Morality." In *Ordinary Ethics: Anthropology, Language, and Action,* edited by Michael Lambek, 368–75. New York: Fordham University Press.

Davidson, Arnold. 2005. "Ethics as Ascetics: Foucault, the History of Ethics, and Ancient Thought." In *The Cambridge Companion to Foucault,* 2nd ed., edited by Gary Gutting, 123–48. Cambridge: Cambridge University Press.

Davis-Floyd, Robbie, and Gloria St. John. 1998. *From Doctor to Healer: The Transformative Journey.* New Brunswick, NJ: Rutgers University Press.

de Certeau, Michel. 1984. *The Practice of Everyday Life.* Berkeley: University of California Press.

Desjarlais, Robert R. 1992. *Body and Emotion: The Aesthetics of Illness and Healing in the Nepal Highlands.* Philadelphia: University of Pennsylvania Press.

———. 1996. "Struggling Along." In *Things as They Are: New Directions in Phenomenological Anthropology,* edited by Michael Jackson, 70–93. Bloomington: Indiana University Press.

———. 1997. *Shelter Blues: Sanity and Selfhood among the Homeless.* Philadelphia: University of Pennsylvania Press.

———. 2003. *Sensory Biographies: Lives and Deaths among Nepal's Yolmo Buddhists.* Berkeley: University of California Press.

Desjarlais, Robert and C.J. Throop. 2011. "Phenomenological Approaches in Anthropology." *Annual Review of Anthropology* 40: 87–102.

Desroche, Henri. 1979. *The Sociology of Hope.* Translated by Carol Martin-Sperry. New York: Routledge.

Dimitriadis, Greg. 2003. *Friendships, Cliques, and Gangs: Young Black Men Coming of Age in Urban America.* New York: Teachers College Press.

Dixon, Patricia. 2009. "Marriage among African Americans: What Does the Research Reveal?" *Journal of African American Studies* 13 (1):29–46.

Dray, William H. 1957. *Laws and Explanations in History.* Oxford: Oxford University Press.

———. 1993. *Philosophy of History.* NJ: Prentice-Hall.

Dreyfus, Hubert, and Paul Rabinow. 1983. *Michel Foucault: Beyond Structuralism and Hermeneutics.* Chicago: University of Chicago Press.

DuBois, W. E. Berghardt. 1903. *The Souls of Black Folk.* Chicago: A.C. McClurg and Co.

DuBois, W. E. Berghardt, and Booker T. Washington. 1903. *The Negro Problem.* Chicago: A.C. McClurg and Co.

Duster, Troy. 2003. *Backdoor to Eugenics,* 2nd ed. New York: Routledge.

———. 2007. *Debating Race: With Michael Eric Dyson.* New York: Basic Civitas.

Ellison, Ralph. 1952. *Invisible Man.* New York: Signet.

Eugene, Toinette M. 1995. "There Is a Balm in Gilead: Black Women and the Black Church as Agents of a Therapeutic Community." *Women and Therapy* 16 (2–3):55–71.

Ewing, Katherine P. 1990. "The Illusion of Wholeness: Culture, Self, and the Experience of Inconsistency." *Ethos* 18 (3):251–78.

Fabian, Johannes. 1983. *Time and the Other: How Anthropology Makes Its Object*. New York: Columbia University Press.

Farran, Carol, Olimpia Paun, and Mary Horton Elliot. 2003. "Spirituality in Multicultural Caregivers of Persons with Dementia." *Dementia* 2 (3):353–77.

Fassin, Didier. 2008. "Beyond Good and Evil? Questioning the Anthropological Discomfort with Morals." *Anthropological Theory* 8 (4):333–44.

———. 2011. *Humanitarian Reason: A Moral History of the Present*. Berkeley: University of California Press.

———. 2014. "Introduction: The Moral Question in Anthropology. In *Moral Anthropology: A Critical Reader*, edited by Didier Fassin and Samuel Leze, 1–16. New York: Routledge.

Faubion, James D. 2001a. "Toward an Anthropology of Ethics: Foucault and the Pedagogies of Autopoiesis." *Representations* 74 (1):83–104.

———. 2001b. *The Ethics of Kinship: Ethnographic Inquiries*. Lanham, MD: Rowman and Littlefield.

———. 2010. "From the Ethical to the Themitical (and Back): Groundwork for an Anthropology of Ethics." In *Ordinary Ethics: Anthropology, Language, and Action*, edited by Michael Lambek, 84–103. New York: Fordham University Press.

———. 2011. *An Anthropology of Ethics*. New York: Cambridge University Press.

Flynn, Thomas. 1997. *Sartre, Foucault, and Historical Reason, Volume One: Toward an Existentialist Theory of History*. Chicago: University of Chicago Press.

Flyvbjerg, Bent. 2001. *Making Social Science Matter: Why Social Inquiry Fails and How It Can Succeed Again*. Translated by Steven Sampson. Cambridge: Cambridge University Press.

Foot, Philippa. 1958. "Moral Beliefs." *Proceedings of the Aristotelian Society* 59:83–104.

Foucault, Michel. 1965. *Madness and Civilization: A History of Insanity in the Age of Reason*. New York: Random House.

———. 1973. *The Birth of the Clinic: An Archaeology of Medical Perception*. New York: Vintage Books.

———. 1979. *Discipline and Punish: The Birth of the Prison*. New York: Vintage Books.

———. 1983. In *Michel Foucault: Beyond Structuralism and Hermeneutics*, edited by Hubert Dreyfus and Paul Rabinow, 232. Chicago: University of Chicago Press.

———. 1990a. *The History of Sexuality, Vol. 1: An Introduction*. Translated by Robert Hurley. New York: Vintage Books.

———. 1990b. *The History of Sexuality, Vol. 2: The Use of Pleasure*. Translated by Robert Hurley. New York: Vintage Books.

———. 1990c. *The History of Sexuality, Volume 3: The Care of the Self*. Translated by Robert Hurley. New York: Vintage Books.

———. 1993. "About the Beginning of the Hermeneutics of the Self: Two Lectures at Dartmouth." *Political Theory* 21 (2):198–227.

———. 1996. In *Foucault Live: Interviews, 1966–84*. Edited by Sylvère Lotringer. Cambridge, MA: MIT Press.

———. 1997a [1984]. "The Ethics of the Concern for Self as a Practice of Freedom." In *Ethics—The Essential Works of Michel Foucault, Vol. 1: Ethics: Subjectivity and Truth,* edited by Paul Rabinow, 281–302. New York: New Press.

———. 1997b [1984]. "Polemics, Politics and Problematizations." In *Ethics— The Essential works of Michel Foucault, Vol. 1: Ethics: Subjectivity and Truth,* edited by Paul Rabinow, 111–20. New York: New Press.

Frank, Arthur W. 1995. *The Wounded Storyteller: Body, Illness, and Ethics.* Chicago: University of Chicago Press.

———. 2010. *Letting Stories Breathe: A Socio-Narratology.* Chicago: University of Chicago Press.

Frankfurt, H. 1971. "Freedom of the Will and the Concept of a Person." *Journal of Philosophy* 68 (1):5–20.

Franklin, Sarah, Jeanette Edwards, Eric Hirsch, Frances Price, and Marilyn Strathern. 1999. *Technologies of Procreation: Kinship in the Age of Assisted Conception.* 2nd edition. New York: Routledge.

Franklin, Sarah, and Margaret Lock. 2003. *Remaking Life and Death.* Santa Fe: School of American Research Press.

Fraser, Gertrude. 1998. *African-American Midwifery in the South: Dialogues of Birth, Race, and Memory.* Cambridge, MA: Harvard University Press.

Frazier, Edward Franklin. 1974 [1963]. *The Negro Church in America.* New York: Schocken.

Freng, Adrienne, and Finn-Aage Esbensen. 2007. "Race and Gang Affiliation: An Examination of Multiple Marginality." *Justice Quarterly* 24 (4):600–628.

Gadamer, Hans Georg. 1973. "Concerning Empty and Ful-filled Time." In *Martin Heidegger: In Europe and America,* edited by Edward Ballard and Charles Scott, 77–89. The Hague: Martinus Nijhoff.

———. 1975. *Truth and Method.* Translated by J. Weinsheimer and D.G. Marshall. New York: Continuum.

———. 1996. *The Enigma of Health: The Art of Healing in a Scientific Age.* Stanford, CA: Stanford University Press.

———. 2004. "A Debate with Hans Georg Gadamer." In *A Ricouer Reader: Reflection and Imagination,* edited by M.J. Valdes. Toronto: University of Toronto Press.

Garcia, Angela. 2010. *The Pastoral Clinic: Addiction and Dispossession along the Rio Grande.* Berkeley: University of California Press.

Gardiner, Michael. 2000. *Critiques of Everyday Life.* New York: Routledge.

Garro, Linda C. 2000. "Cultural Knowledge as Resource in Illness Narratives: Remembering through Accounts of Illness." In *Narrative and the Cultural Construction of Illness and Healing,* edited by Cheryl Mattingly and Linda Garro. 70–87. Berkeley: University of California Press.

———. 2003. Narrating Troubling Experiences. *Transcultural Psychiatry* 40 (1):5–43.

Gates, Henry Jr., and Cornel West. 1996. *The Future of the Race.* New York: Knopf.

Geertz, Clifford. 1973. *The Interpretation of Cultures.* New York: Basic Books.

———. 1983. *Local Knowledge: Further Essays in Interpretive Anthropology.* New York: Basic Books.

Gilroy, Paul. 1993. *The Black Atlantic: Modernity and Double Consciousness.* Cambridge, MA: Harvard University Press.

Goldberg, David Theo. 1997. *Racial Subjects: Writing on Race in America.* New York: Routledge.

Good, Byron. 1994. *Medicine, Rationality, and Experience: An Anthropological Perspective.* New York: Cambridge University Press.

Good, Mary-Jo DelVecchio. 2007. "The Medical Imaginary and the Biotechnical Embrace: Subjective Experiences of Clinical Scientists and Patients." In *Subjectivity: Ethnographic Investigations,* edited by Joao Biehl, Byron Good, and Arthur Kleinman, 362–80. Berkeley: University of California Press.

———. 1995. *American Medicine: The Quest for Competence.* Berkeley: University of California Press.

Good, Mary-Jo DelVecchio, Sarah Willen, Seth Donal, Hannah, Ken Vickory, and Lawrence Taeseng Park, eds. 2011. *Shattering Culture: American Medicine Responds to Cultural Diversity.* New York: Russell Sage Foundation.

Goodwin, Marjorie. 1990. *He-Said-She-Said: Talk as Social Organization among Black Children.* Bloomington: Indiana University Press.

———. 2007. "Occasioned Knowledge Exploration in Family Interaction." *Discourse and Society* 18 (1): 93–110.

Grant, Jacquelyn. 1989. "Womanist Theology: Black Women's Experience as a Source for Doing Theology with Special Reference to Christology." In *African American Religious Studies: An Interdisciplinary Anthology,* edited by Gayraud Wilmore, 208–27. Durham, NC: Duke University Press.

Grøn, Lone. 2005. "Winds of Change, Bodies of Persistence." Doctoral Dissertation, University of Aarhus, Denmark.

Grøn, Lone, Cheryl Mattingly, and Lotte Meinert. 2008. "Kronisk hjemmearbejde: Sociale hab, dilemmaer og konflikter I hjemmearbejdnarrativer i Uganda, danmark og USA." [Chronic Homework: Social Hopes, Dilemmas, and Conflicts in Homework Narratives in Uganda, Denmark, and the USA] *Tidsskrift for forskning I sygdom og samfund* 9: 71–96.

Guignon, Charles. 2009. "Williams and the Phenomenological Tradition." In *Reading Bernard Williams,* edited by Daniel Callcut, 189–210. New York: Routledge.

Gutting, Gary., ed. 2005. *The Cambridge Companion to Foucault,* 2nd ed. Cambridge: Cambridge University Press.

Hanne, Michael. 2010. "Narrative and Metaphor in Medicine: An Overview." *Genre* 44 (3):223–37.

Hannerz, Ulf. 1969. *Soulside: Inquiries into Ghetto Culture and Community.* New York: Columbia University Press.

Harmon, Julia Robinson. 2006. "The Leadership of Reverend Robert L. Bradby and the Black Community in East Industrial Detroit." In *The Black Urban Community: From Dusk Till Dawn,* edited by Gayle Tate and Lewis Randolph, 204–226. New York: Palgrave Macmillan.

Harvey, David. 2000. *Spaces of Hope.* Berkeley: University of California Press.

Hebert, Randy, Molly Jenckes, Daniel Ford, Debra O'Connor, and Lisa Cooper. 2001. "Patient Perspectives on Spirituality and the Patient-Physician Relationship." *Journal of General Internal Medicine* 16 (10):685–92.

Heidegger, Martin. 1962. *Being and Time*. Translated by John Macquarrie and Edward Robinson. London: SCM.

Hempel, Carl G. 1942. "The Function of General Laws in History." *Journal of Philosophy* 39 (2):35–48.

Hicks, H. Beecher Jr. 1994. "Challenge to the African American Church: Problems and Perspectives for the Third Millennium." *Journal of Religious Thought* 51 (1):81.

Hine, Darlene, and Kathleen Thompson. 1998. *A Shining Thread of Hope*. New York: Broadway Books.

Hines, Paulette Moore, and Nancy Boyd–Franklin. 1996. "African American Families." In *Ethnicity and Family Therapy*, 2nd Edition, edited by Monica McGoldrick, Joe Giordano, and John Pearce, 66–84. London: Guilford.

hooks, bell. 1990. "Postmodern Blackness." *Postmodern Culture* 1 (1).

———. 1992. *Black Looks: Race and Representation*. Boston: South End Press.

———. 1994. *Outlaw Culture: Resisting Representations*. New York: Routledge.

———. 1995. *Killing Rage: Ending Racism*. New York: Henry Holt & Co.

Hollan, Douglas. 2012. "On the Varieties and Particularities of Cultural Experience." *Ethos* 40 (1):37–53.

Holland, Dorothy, William Lachicotte Jr. and Carole Cain. 1998/2001. *Identity and Agency in Cultural Works*. Cambridge, MA: Harvard University Press.

Howell, James, Arlen Egley Jr., George Tita, and Elizabeth Griffiths. 2011. "U.S. Gang Problems and Seriousness, 1996–2009." *National Gang Center Bulletin*, No. 6. http://www.nationalgangcenter.gov/content/documents/bulletin-6.pdf.

Howell, Signe. 1997. *The Ethnography of Moralities*. Oxford: Taylor & Francis.

Huff, C. Ronald, ed. 2008. "Gang Violence." In *Encyclopedia of Interpersonal Violence*, 289–91. Thousand Oaks, CA: SAGE. *SAGE Reference Online*.

Hughes, Langston. 1994. "Dreams." In *The Collected Poems of Langston Hughes*, edited by Arnold Rampersad and David Roessel, 32. New York: Knopf.

Hughes, Lorine, and James Short. 2005. "Disputes Involving Youth Street Gang Members: Micro-Social Contexts*." *Criminology* 43 (1):43–76.

Humphrey, Caroline. 2008. "Reassembling Individual Subjects: Events and Decisions in Troubled Times." *Anthropological Theory* 8 (4):357–80.

Hunter, Andrea. 1997. "Counting on Grandmothers: Black Mothers' and Fathers' Reliance on Black Grandmothers for Parenting." *Journal of Family Issues* 18 (3):251–69.

Hunter, Kathryn. 1991. *Doctors' Stories: The Narrative Structure of Medical Knowledge*. Princeton: Princeton University Press.

Hursthouse, Rosalind. 1999. *On Virtue Ethics*. New York: Oxford University Press.

Hutson, H. Range, Deirdre Anglin, and Michael Pratts Jr. 1994. "Adolescents and Children Injured or Killed in Drive-By Shootings in Los Angeles." *New England Journal of Medicine* 330 (5):324–27.

Hyland, Drew, and John Manoussakis. 2006. *Heidegger and the Greeks: Interpretive Essays*. Bloomington: Indiana University Press.

Iser, Wolfgang. 1980. *The Act of Reading: A Theory of Aesthetic Response*. Baltimore: John Hopkins University Press.

Jackson, Michael. 1989. *Paths toward a Clearing: Radical Empiricism and Ethnographic Inquiry.* Bloomington: Indiana University Press.

———. 1995. *At Home in the World.* Durham, NC: Duke University Press.

———. 1996, ed. *Things As They Are: New Directions in Phenomenological Anthropology.* Bloomington: Indiana University Press.

———. 2002. *The Politics of Storytelling: Violence, Transgression, and Intersubjectivity.* Copenhagen: University of Copenhagen Press.

———. 2005. *Existential Anthropology: Events, Exigencies and Effects: Methodology and History in Anthropology Vol. 11.* Oxford: Berghahn.

———, ed. 2007. *Excursions.* Durham, NC: Duke University Press.

Jacobs, Lanita, Mary Lawlor, and Cheryl Mattingly. 2011. "I/We Narratives among African American Families Raising Children with Special Needs." *Culture, Medicine, and Psychiatry* 35 (1):3–25.

Jacobs, Ronald. 2000. *Race, Media, and the Crisis of Civil Society: From Watts to Rodney King.* Cambridge: Cambridge University Press.

Jarrett, Robin. 1995. "Growing Up Poor: The Family Experiences of Socially Mobile Youth in Low-Income African American Neighborhoods." *Journal of Adolescent Research* 10 (1):111–35.

Jay, Martin. 2005. *Songs of Experience: Modern American and European Variations on a Universal Theme.* Berkeley: University of California Press.

Jimerson, Jason, and Matthew Oware. 2006. "Telling the Code of the Street: An Ethnomethodological Ethnography." *Journal of Contemporary Ethnography* 35 (1):24–50.

Jordan, Brigitte. 1978. *Birth in Four Cultures: A Crosscultural Investigation of Childbirth in Yucatan, Holland, Sweden, and the United States.* Prospect Heights, IL: Waveland.

———. 1989. "Cosmopolitical Obstetrics: Some Insights from the Training of Traditional Midwives." *Social Science and Medicine* 28 (9):925–44.

———. 1997. "Authoritative Knowledge and Its Construction." In *Childbirth and Authoritative Knowledge: Cross-Cultural Perspectives,* edited by Robbie Davis-Floyd and Carolyn Sargent, 55–79. Berkeley: University of California Press.

Keane, Webb. 2007. *Christian Moderns: Freedom and Fetish in the Mission Encounter.* Berkeley: University of California Press.

———. 2010. "Minds, Surfaces, and Reasons in the Anthropology of Ethics." In *Ordinary Ethics: Anthropology, Language, and Action,* edited by Michael Lambek, 64–83. New York: Fordham University Press.

Kelch-Oliver, Karla. 2011. "The Experiences of African American Grandmothers in Grandparent-Headed Families." *Family Journal* 19 (1):73–82.

King, Sharon. 1998. "The Beam in Thine Own Eye: Disability and the Black Church." *Western Journal of Black Studies* 22 (1):37–48.

Kleinman, Arthur. 1989. *The Illness Narratives: Suffering, Healing, and the Human Condition.* New York: Basic Books.

———. 1999a. "Experience and Its Moral Modes: Culture, Human Condition, and Disorder." In *The Tanner Lectures on Human Values,* Vol. 20, edited by G. B. Peterson, 357–420. Salt Lake City: University of Utah Press.

———. 1999b. "Moral Experience and Ethical Reflection: Can Ethnography Reconcile Them? A Quandy for 'The New Bioethics.'" *Daedalus* 128 (4):69–97.

———. 2006. *What Really Matters: Living a Moral Life amidst Uncertainty and Danger*. Oxford: Oxford University Press.

Kleinman, Arthur, and Joan Kleinman. 1991. "Suffering and Its Professional Transformation: Toward an Ethnography of Interpersonal Experience." *Culture, Medicine and Psychiatry* 15 (3):275–301.

Kleinman, Arthur, Veena Das, and Margaret Lock. 1997. *Social Suffering*. Berkeley: University of California Press.

Knight, Kelvin. 2007. *Aristotelian Philosophy: Ethics and Politics from Aristotle to MacIntyre*. Cambridge: Polity Press.

Kremer-Sadlik, Tamar, and Jeemin Lydia Kim. 2007. "Lessons from Sports: Children's Socialization to Values through family Interaction during Sports Activities." *Discourse and Society* 18 (1):35–52.

Labov, William. 1972. *Language in the Inner City: Studies in the Black English Vernacular*. Philadelphia: University of Pennsylvania Press.

Laidlaw, James. 2002. "For an Anthropology of Ethics and Freedom." *Journal of the Royal Anthropological Institute* 8 (2):311–32.

———. 2010. "Agency and Responsibility: Perhaps You Can Have Too Much of a Good Thing." In *Ordinary Ethics: Anthropology, Language, and Action*, edited by Michael Lambek, 143–64. New York: Fordham University Press.

———. 2013. *The Subject of Virtue: An Anthropology of Ethics and Freedom*. Cambridge: Cambridge University Press.

Lakoff, George, and Mark Johnson. 1980. *Metaphors We Live By*. Chicago: University of Chicago Press.

Lambek, Michael. 1996. "The Past Imperfect: Remembering as Moral Practice." In *Tense Past: Cultural Essays in Trauma and Memory*, edited by Paul Antze and Michael Lambek, 235–54. New York: Routledge.

———. 2000. "The Anthropology of Religion and the Quarrel between Poetry and Philosophy." *Current Anthropology* 41 (3):309–20.

———. 2002a. *The Weight of the Past: Living with History in Mahajanga, Madagascar*. New York: Palgrave Macmillan.

———. 2002b. "Fantasy in Practice: Projection and Introjection, or the Witch and the Spirit-Medium." *Social analysis* 46 (3):198–214.

———. 2003. "Introduction: Irony and Illness—Recognition and Refusal." *Social Analysis* 47 (2), 1–19.

———. 2008. "Value and Virtue." *Anthropological Theory* 8 (2):133–57.

———. 2010a. "Toward and Ethics of the Act." In *Ordinary Ethics: Anthropology, Language, and Action*, edited by Michael Lambek, 39–63. New York: Fordham University Press.

———, 2010b. "Introduction." In *Ordinary Ethics: Anthropology, Language, and Action*, edited by Michael Lambek, 1–36. New York: Fordham University Press.

———. 2013. "The Continuous and Discontinuous Person: Two Dimensions of Ethical Life." *Journal of the Royal Anthropological Institute* 19(4):837–58.

Latour, Bruno, Steve Wolgaar, and Jonas Salk. 1979. *Laboratory Life: The Social Construction of Scientific Facts*. Thousand Oaks, CA: Sage.

Lawlor, Mary C. 2003. "The Significance of Being Occupied: The Social Construction of Childhood." *American Journal of Occupational Therapy* 57 (4):424–434

———. 2004. "Mothering Work: Negotiating Healthcare, Illness and Disability, and Development." In *Mothering Occupations,* edited by Susan Esdaile and J. Olson, 306–323. Philadelphia: F. A. Davis.

———. 2012. "The Particularities of Engagement." *Occupational Therapy Journal of Research* 32(4): 131–159.

———. 2006. *Radical Hope: Ethics in the Face of Cultural Devastation.* Cambridge, MA: Harvard University Press.

Lear, Jonathan. 2000. *Happiness, Death, and the Remainder of Life.* Cambridge, MA: Harvard University Press.

Lempert, Lora. 1999. "Other Fathers: An Alternative Perspective on African American Community Caring." In *The Black Family: Essays and Studies,* 6th ed., edited by Robert Staples, 189–201. Belmont, CA: Wadsworth.

Levin, Jeffrey, and Robert Taylor. 1997. "Age Differences in the Patterns and Correlates of the Frequency of Prayer." *Gerontologist* 37 (1):75–88.

Levin, Jeffrey, Robert Taylor, and Linda Chatters. 1994. "Race and Gender Differences in Religiosity among Older Adults: Findings from Four National Surveys." *Journal of Gerontology: Social Sciences* 49 (3):137–45.

Linger, Daniel. 1994. "Has Culture Theory Lost Its Minds?" *Ethos* 22 (3):284–315.

Luhrmann, Tanya M. 2006. "Subjectivity." *Anthropological Theory* 6 (3):345–61.

———. 2012. When God Talks Back. New York: Random House.

Lyotard, Jean.1979. *The Postmodern Condition: A Report on Knowledge,* Vol. 10. Minneapolis: University of Minnesota Press.

MacIntyre, Alasdaire. 1981. *After Virtue: A Study in Moral Theory.* Notre Dame, IN: University of Notre Dame Press.

———. 1988. *Whose Justice, Which Rationality?* Notre Dame, IN: University of Notre Dame Press.

———. 1990. *Three Rival Versions of Moral Inquiry.* Notre Dame, IN: University of Notre Dame Press.

———. 2001. *Dependent Rational Animals: Why Human Beings Need the Virtues.* Chicago: Open Court.

Mahmood, Saba. 2005. *Politics of Piety: The Islamic Revival and the Feminist Subject.* Princeton: Princeton University Press.

Mansfield, Christopher, Jim Mitchell, and Dana King. 2002. "The Doctor as God's Mechanic? Beliefs in the Southeastern United States." *Social Science and Medicine* 54 (3):399–409.

Markens, Susan, Sarah Fox, Bonnie Taub, and Mary Lou Gilbert. 2002. "Role of Black Churches in Health Promotion Programs: Lessons from the Los Angeles Mammography Promotion in Churches Program." *American Journal of Public Health* 92 (5):805–10.

Martin, Emily. 1987. *The Woman in the Body.* Boston: Beacon.

———. 1994. *Flexible Bodies: Tracking Immunity in American Culture from the Days of Polio to the Days of AIDS.* Boston: Beacon.

Marx, Karl, and Friedrich Engels. 2002 [1845]. *The Holy Family.* Honolulu: University Press of the Pacific.

———. 2004 [1852]. *The Eighteenth Brumaire of Louis Bonaparte.* Whitefish, UK: Kessinger.

Matthews, Holly F., Donald R. Lannin, and James P. Mitchell. 1994. "Coming to Terms with Advanced Breast Cancer: Black Women's Narratives from Eastern North Carolina." *Social Science and Medicine* 38 (6):798–800.

Mattingly, Cheryl. 1998a. "In Search of the Good: Narrative Reasoning in Clinical Practice." *Medical Anthropology Quarterly* 12 (3):273–97.

———. 1998b. *Healing Dramas and Clinical Plots: The Narrative Structure of Experience.* Cambridge: Cambridge University Press.

———. 2000. "Emergent Narratives." In *Narrative and the Cultural Construction of Illness and Healing,* edited by Cheryl Mattingly and Linda Garro, 181–210. Berkeley: University of California Press.

———. 2006a. "Reading Medicine: Mind, Body, and Meditation in One Interpretive Community." *New Literary History* 37 (3):563–81.

———. 2006b. "Suffering and Narrative Re-envisioning." *Hedgehog Review: Critical Reflections on Contemporary Culture* 8 (3):21–35.

———. 2009. "Senses of an Ending: Self, Body and Narrative." In *Narrative, Self and Social Practice,* edited by Uffe Juul Jensen and Cheryl Mattingly, 245–269. Aarhus: Philosophia Press.

———. 2010a. "Moral Willing as Narrative Re-envisioning." In *Towards an Anthropology of the Will,* edited by Keith Murphy and Jason Throop, 50–69. Stanford, CA: Stanford University Press.

———. 2010b. *The Paradox of Hope: Journeys through a Clinical Borderland.* Berkeley: University of California Press.

———. 2011. "The Machine-Body as Contested Metaphor in Clinical Care." *Genre: Forms of Discourse and Culture.* Special Issue: *Binocular Vision: Narrative and Metaphor in Medicine* 44 (3):363–80.

———. 2012. "Two Virtue Ethics and the Anthropology of Morality." *Anthropology Theory* 12 (2):161–84.

———. 2013. "Moral Selves and Moral Scenes: Narrative Experiments in Everyday Life." *Ethnos* 78 (3):301–27.

———. 2014. "The Moral Perils of a Superstrong Black Mother." *Ethos* 42(1):119–138.

———. In Press, a. "Love's Imperfection: Moral Becoming, Friendship and Family Life." *Suomen Antropologi (Finnish Journal of Anthropology).* Special Issue: *The Morality of Friendship.* James Throop and Valerio Simoni, guest editors.

———. In Press, b. "'Turn Your Fear Into Fire': An Uneasy Experiment in Radical Cultural Comparison – Los Angeles Gangs and the Moral Universe of Marquis de Sade. *Ethnos.*

———. In Press, c. "Moral Deliberation and the Agentive Self in Laidlaw's Ethics." *HAU Journal of Ethnographic Theory.*

Mattingly, Cheryl, Lone Grøn, and Lotte Meinert. 2011. "Chronic Homework in Emerging Borderlands of Healthcare." *Culture, Medicine and Psychiatry* 35 (3):347–75.

Mattingly, Cheryl, Uffe Jensen, and Jason Throop. 2009. "Narrative, Self and Social Practice." In *Narrative, Self and Social Practice,* edited by Uffe Jensen and Cheryl Mattingly, 1–36. Aarhus: Philosophia Press.

Mattingly, Cheryl and Uffe Jensen. In Press. "What Can We Hope For? An Exploration in Cosmopolitan Philosophical Anthropology." In *Anthropol-*

ogy & Philosophy: Dialogues on Trust and Hope, edited by S. Liisberg, E. Pedersen, and A. Dalsgård. Oxford: Berghahn.

Mbembe, Achille. 1992. "The Banality of Power and the Aesthetics of Vulgarity in the Postcolony." *Public Culture* 4 (2):1–30.

Mbiti, John. 1969. *African Religions and Philosophy*. New York: Praeger.

Meehan, Patrick, and Patrick O'Carroll. 1992. "Gangs, Drugs, and Homicide in Los Angeles." *Archives of Pediatrics and Adolescent Medicine* 146(6): 683–87.

Mhyre, Knut. 1998. "The Anthropological Concept of Action and Its Problems: A 'New' Approach Based on Marcel Mauss and Aristotle." *Journal of the Anthropological Society of Oxford*. 29:121–34.

Miles, Tiya. 2008. "The Black Mother Within." *Black Women, Gender and Families* 2 (2):99–103.

Minkler, Meredith, and Kathleen Roe. 1993. *Grandmothers as Caregivers: Raising Children of the Crack Cocaine Epidemic*. Newbury Park, CA: Sage.

Miyazaki, Hirokazu. 2004. *The Method of Hope: Anthropology, Philosophy, and Fijian Knowledge*. Stanford, CA: Stanford University Press.

Moody-Adams, Michele. 1997. *Fieldwork in Familiar Places. Morality, Culture, and Philosophy*. Cambridge, MA: Harvard University Press.

Morgan Quinto Corporation. 2006. *City Crime Rankings*. Lawrence, KS: Morgan Quinto.

Morrison, Toni. 1987. *Beloved*. New York: Knopf.

———. 1997. *Paradise*. New York: Knopf.

Murdoch, Iris. 1970. *The Sovereignty of Good*. New York: Ark Paperbacks.

Murphy, Keith and Jason Throop, eds. 2010. *Toward an Anthropology of the Will*. Stanford, CA: Stanford University Press.

Myrics, Orlando, and Clifford Jordan. 2007, February. *Why We Bang—A Film on Bloods and Crips in Los Angeles*, Part 1. Documentary, 9:41 minutes. http://www.youtube.com/watch?v = O2x4KAAN27k.

———. 2007, February. *Why We Bang—A Film on Bloods and Crips in Los Angeles*, Part 2. Documentary, 9:26 minutes. http://www.youtube.com /watch?v = VnRJ3j1SSpM.

Nadasen, Premilla. 2007. "From Widow to 'Welfare Queen.'" *Black Women, Gender and Families* 1 (2):52–77.

National Drug Intelligence Center. 2007, June. "Drug Trafficking Organizations." In *Los Angeles High Intensity Drug Trafficking Area Drug Market Analysis*, Document ID: 2007-R0813–013. http://www.justice.gov/archive /ndic/pubs23/23937/dtos.htm.

Navaie-Waliser, Maryam, Penny Feldman, David Gould, Carol Levine, Alexis Kuerbis, and Karen Donelan. 2001. "The Experiences and Challenges of Informal Caregivers: Common Themes and Differences among Whites, Blacks, and Hispanics." *Gerontologist* 41 (6):1–9.

Nehamas, Alexander. 1998. *The Art of Living*. Berkeley: University of California Press.

Ness, Cindy D. 2010. *Why Girls Fight: Female Youth Violence in the Inner City*. New York: New York University Press.

Nightingale, Marcie C. 2003. "Religion, Spirituality, and Ethnicity: What It Means for Caregivers of Persons with Alzheimer's Disease and Related Disorders." *Dementia* 2 (3):379–91.

Noddings, Nell. 1984. *Caring: A Feminine Approach to Ethics and Moral Education*. Berkeley: University of California Press.

Nussbaum, Martha. 1986. *The Fragility of Goodness: Luck and Ethics in Greek Tragedy and Philosophy*. New York: Cambridge University Press.

———. 1990. *Love's Knowledge: Essays on Philosophy and Literature*. Oxford: Oxford University Press.

———. 1993. "Non-Relative Virtues: An Aristotelion Approach." In *The Quality of Life*, edited by Martha Nussbaum and Amartya Sen, 242–69. Oxford: Oxford University Press.

———. 1994. *The Therapy of Desire: Theory and Practice in Hellenistic Ethics*. Princeton: Princeton University Press.

———. 1999. "Virtue Ethics: A Misleading Category?" *Journal of Ethics* 3: 163–201.

———. 2001. *Upheavals of Thought: The Intelligence of Emotions*. Cambridge: Cambridge University Press.

———. 2009. "Bernard Williams: Tragedies, Hope, Justice." In *Reading Bernard Williams*, edited by Daniel Callcut, 213–41. New York: Routledge.

Nussbaum, Martha, and Amartya Sen, eds. 1999. *The Quality of Life*. New York: Oxford University Press.

Ochs, Elinor. 1988. *Culture and Language Development: Language Acquisition and Language Socialization in a Samoan Village*. Cambridge: Cambridge University Press.

Ochs, Elinor, and Lisa Capps. 2001. *Living Narrative: Creating Lives in Everyday Storytelling*. Cambridge, MA: Harvard University Press.

Ochs, Elinor, and Tamar Kremer-Sadlik. 2007. "Introduction: Morality as Family Practice." *Discourse and Society* 18 (1):5–10.

Okazawa-Rey, Margo. 1994. "Grandparents Who Care: An Empowerment Model of Health Care." In *"It Just Ain't Fair": The Ethics of Health Care of African Americans*, edited by Annette Dula and Sara Goering, 221–33. New York: Praeger.

Olafson, Frederick. 1979. *The Dialectic of Action: A Philosophical Interpretation of History and the Humanities*. Chicago: University of Chicago Press.

Oliver, William. 2006. "'The Streets': An Alternative Black Male Socialization Institution." *Journal of Black Studies* 36 (6):918–37.

Ong, Aihwa and Stephen Collier, eds. 2008. *Global Assemblages: Technology, Politics, and Ethics as Anthropological Problems*. Malden, MA: Blackwell.

Ortner, Sherry. 2005. "Subjectivity and Cultural Critique." *Anthropological Theory* 5 (1):31–52.

Papachristos, Andrew. 2009. "Murder by Structure: Dominance Relations and the Social Structure of Gang Homicide." *American Journal of Sociology* 115 (1):74–128.

Paras, Eric. 2006. *Foucault 2.0: Beyond Power and Knowledge*. New York: Other Press.

Parish, Steven. 1994. *Moral Knowing in a Hindu Sacred City: An Exploration of Mind, Emotion, and Self*. New York: Columbia University Press.

Pattillo-McCoy, Mary. 1998. "Church Culture as a Strategy of Action in the Black Community." *American Sociological Review* 63 (6):767–84.

Petersen, Alan. 2003. "Governmentality, Critical Scholarship, and the Medical Humanities." *Journal of Medical Humanities* 24 (3–4):187–201.

Poindexter, Cynthia, and Nathan Linsk. 1999. "'I'm Just Glad That I'm Here': Stories of Seven African-American HIV-Affected Grandmothers." *Journal of Gerontological Social Work* 32 (1):63–81.

Polzer, Rebecca, and Margaret Miles. 2005. "Spirituality and Self-Management of Diabetes in African Americans." *Journal of Holistic Nursing* 23 (2):230–50.

Potts, Randolph. 1996. "Spirituality and the Experience of Cancer in an African-American Community: Implications of Psychosocial Oncology." *Journal of Psychosocial Oncology* 14 (1):1–19.

Powell, Jason, and Simon Biggs. 2004. "Ageing, Technologies of Self and Bio-Medicine: A Foucauldian Excursion." *International Journal of Sociology and Social Policy* 24 (6):17–29.

Rabinow, Paul, ed. 1984a. *The Foucault Reader*. New York: Pantheon.

———. 1984b. *Ethics—The Essential works of Michel Foucault, Vol. 1: Ethics: Subjectivity and Truth*, edited by Paul Rabinow, 111–20. New York: New Press.

———. 1996a. *Essays on the Anthropology of Reason*. Princeton: Princeton University Press.

———. 1996b. *Making PCR: A Story of Biotechnology*. Chicago: University of Chicago Press.

Radin, Paul. 1957 [1927]. *Primitive Man as Philosopher*. New York: Schocken.

Rapp, Rayna, and Faye Ginsburg. 2001. "Enabling Disability: Rewriting Kinship, Reimagining Citizenship." *Public Culture* 13 (3):533–56.

Read, Kenneth. 1955. "Morality and the Concept of the Person among the Gahuku-Gama." *Oceania*, 25: 233–82.

Renzetti, Claire and Jeffrey L. Edleson, eds. 2008. "Gang Violence." In *Encyclopedia of Interpersonal Violence*, 288–90. Los Angeles: Sage.

Reverby, Susan. 2000. *Tuskegee's Truths: Rethinking the Tuskegee Syphilis Study*. Chapel Hill: University of North Carolina Press.

Richardson, Marilyn. 1980. *Black Women and Religion: A Bibliography*. Boston: GK Hall Co.

Ricoeur, Paul. 1978. *The Philosophy of Paul Ricoeur: An Anthology of His Work*, edited by Charles Reagan and David Stewart. Boston: Beacon Press.

———. 1981. *Paul Ricoeur: Hermeneutics and the Human Sciences: Essays on Language, Action, and Interpretation*, edited by John Thompson. Cambridge: Cambridge University Press.

———. 1984. *Time and Narrative*, vol. 1. Translated by Kathleen McLaughlin and David Pellauer. Chicago: University of Chicago Press.

———. 1985. *Time and Narrative*, vol. 2. Translated by Kathleen McLaughlin and David Pellauer. Chicago: University of Chicago Press.

———. 1988. *Time and Narrative*, vol. 3. Translated by Kathleen Blamey and David Pellauer. Chicago: University of Chicago Press.

———. 1992. *Oneself as Another*. Translated by Kathleen Blamey. Chicago: University of Chicago Press.

Roberts, Dorothy. 1998. "The Absent Black Father." In *Lost Fathers: The politics of fatherlessness in America*, edited by Cynthia Daniels, 45–162. New York: St. Martins.

Robbins, Joel. 2004. *Becoming Sinners: Christianity and Moral Torment in a Papua New Guinea Society*. Berkeley: University of California Press.

———. 2007. "Between Reproduction and Freedom: Morality, Value, and Radical Cultural Change." *Ethnos* 72 (3):293–314.

———. 2009. "Value, Structure and the Range of Possibilities: A Response to Zigon." *Ethnos* 74:277–85.

———. 2013. "Beyond the Suffering Subject: Toward an Anthropology of the Good." *Journal of the Royal Anthropological Institute* 19(3): 447–62.

Rogers-Dulan, Jeanette, and Jan Blacher. 1995. "African American Families, Religion, and Disability: A Conceptual Framework." *Mental Retardation* 33 (4):226–38.

Rosaldo, Renato. 1984. "Grief and a Headhunter's Rage: On the Cultural Force of Emotions." In *Text, Play, and Story: The Construction and Reconstruction of Self and Society*, edited by Stuart Bruner and Edward Plattner, 178–95. Washington, DC: American Ethnological Society.

———. 1989. *Culture and Truth: The Remaking of Social Analysis*. Boston: Beacon Press.

Rose, Nikolas. 1990. *Governing the Soul: The Shaping of the Private Self*. London: Routledge.

———. 1998. *Inventing Our Selves: Psychology, Power, and Personhood*. Cambridge: Cambridge University Press.

———. 2007. *The Politics of Life Itself: Biomedicine, Power, and Subjectivity in the Twenty First Century*. Princeton: Princeton University Press.

Rouse, Carolyn. 2004. "'If She's a Vegetable, We'll Be Her Garden': Embodiment, Transcendence, and Citations of Competing Cultural Metaphors in the Case of a Dying Child." *American Ethnologist* 31 (4):514–29.

Rouse, Carolyn. 2009. *Uncertain Suffering: Racial Health Care Disparities and Sickle Cell Disease*. Berkeley: University of California Press.

Ruble, Nikki, and William Turner. 2000. "A System Analysis of the Dynamics and Organization of Urban Street Gangs." *American Journal of Family Therapy* 28: 117–32.

Sahlins, Marshall David. 1995. *How "Natives" Think: About Captain Cook, for Example*. Chicago: University of Chicago Press.

Sanders, Jo-Ann, and Carla Bradley. 2005. "Multiple-Lens Paradigm: Evaluating African American Girls and Their Development." *Journal of Counseling and Development* 83 (3):292–98.

Scheper-Hughes, Nancy. 1993. *Death without Weeping: The Violence of Everyday Life in Brazil*. Berkeley: University of California Press.

Schneewind, Jerome. 1998. *The Invention of Autonomy: A History of Modern Moral Philosophy*. Cambridge: Cambridge University Press.

Schön, Donald. 1979. "Generative Metaphor: A Perspective on Problem-Setting in Social Policy." In *Metaphor and Thought*, edited by Andrew Ortony, 137–63. Cambridge: Cambridge University Press.

Seaton, Eleanor, and Ronald Taylor. 2003. "Exploring Familial Processes in Urban, Low-Income African American Families." *Journal of Family Issues* 24 (5):627–44.

Sharp, Elizabeth, and Jean Ipsa. 2009. "Inner City Single Black Mothers' Gender-Related Childrearing Expectations and Goals." *Sex Roles* 60 (9–10):656–68.

Sherry, Alissa, Keith Wood, Emily Jackson, and Nadine Kaslow. 2006. "Racist Events and Ethnic Identity in Low Income, African Americans." *Journal of Applied Social Psychology* 36 (6):1365–80.

Sistler, Audrey, and Kimberly Washington. 1999. "Serenity for African American Caregivers." *Social Work with Groups* 22 (1):49–62.

Smitherman, Gene. 1999. *Talking that Talk: Language, Culture and Education in African America*. New York: Routledge.

Staples, Robert. 1999. "The Dyad." In *The Black Family: Essays and Studies*, 6th ed., edited by Robert Staples, 40–44. Belmont, CA: Wadsworth.

Stewart, Carlyle Fielding III. 1997. *Soul Survivors: An African American spirituality*. Louisville: Westminster.

Stoczkowski, Wiktor. 2008. The "Fourth Aim" of Anthropology: Between Knowledge and Ethics. *Anthropological Theory* 8: 345–56.

Taylor, Carl, Richard Lerner, Alexander von Eye, Deborah Bobek, Aida Bilalbegovic Balsano, Elizabeth Dowling, and Pamela Anderson. 2005. "Internal and External Developmental Assets among African American Male Gang Members." *Journal of Adolescent Research* 19 (3):303–22.

Taylor, Carl, Richard Lerner, Alexander von Eye, Deborah Bobek, Aida Balsano, Elizabeth Dowling, and Pamela Anderson. 2003. "Positive Individual and Social Behavior among Gang and Nongang African American Male Adolescents." *Journal of Adolescent Research* 18 (5):496–522.

Taylor, Charles. 1964. *The Explanation of Behaviour*. New York: Routledge.

———. 1985. "Connolly, Foucault, and Truth." *Political Theory* 13 (3):377–85.

———. 1989. *Sources of the Self*. Cambridge, MA: Harvard University Press.

———. 2007. *A Secular Age*. Cambridge, MA: Harvard University Press.

Taylor, Janelle, 2005. "Surfacing the Body Interior." *Annual Review of Anthropology* 34:741–756.

Taylor, Robert, Christopher Ellison, Linda Chatters, Jeffrey Levin, and Karen Lincoln. 2000. "Mental Health Services in Faith Communities: The Role of Clergy in Black Churches." *Social Work* 45 (1):73–87.

Thompson, John. 1984. *Critical Hermeneutics: A Study in the Thought of Paul Ricoeur and Jürgen Habermas*. Cambridge: Cambridge University Press.

Throop, Jason. 2003. "Articulating Experience." *Anthropological Theory* 3 (1):2–26.

———. 2009. "Intermediary Varieties of Experience." *Ethnos* 74: 535–58.

———. 2010a. "In the Midst of Action." In *Toward an Anthropology of the Will*, edited by Keith Murphy and Jason Throop, 28–49. Stanford, CA: Stanford University Press.

———. 2010b. *Suffering and Sentiment: Exploring the Vicissitudes of Experience and Pain in Yap*. Berkeley: University of California Press.

Tronto, Joan. 1993. *Moral Boundaries: A Political Argument for an Ethic of Care*. London: Routledge.

Turner, Victor. 1986. "Dewey, Dilthey, and Drama: An Essay in the Anthropology of Experience." In *The Anthropology of Experience*, edited by Victor Turner and Edward Bruner, 33–44. Chicago: University of Illinois Press.

Turner, Victor, and Edward Bruner, eds. 1986. *The Anthropology of Experience*. Chicago: University of Illinois Press.

United States Congress Proceedings. 2006. "Combating Youth Violence: What Federal, State and Local Governments Are Doing to Deter Youth Crime."

Valentine, Daniel E. 1996. *Charred Lullabies: Chapters in an Anthropography of Violence*. Princeton: Princeton University Press.

Vargas, Joao H. Costa. 2006. *Catching Hell in the City of Angels: Life and Meanings of Blackness in South Central Los Angeles*. Minneapolis: University of Minnesota Press.

Vigil, James Diego. 2003. "Urban Violence and Street Gangs." *Annual Review of Anthropology* 32: 225–42.

Villaraigosa, Antonio R. 2007, April 18. "City of Los Angeles Gang Reduction Strategy." http://file.lacounty.gov/bos/supdocs/32068.pdf.

Vogel, Shane. 2009. "By the Light of What Comes After: Eventologies of the Ordinary." *Women and Performance: A Journal of Feminist Theory* 19 (2):247–63.

Wacquant, Loic. 2008. *Urban Outcasts: A Comparative Sociology of Advanced Marginality*. Malden, MA: Polity Press.

Waite, Maurice, ed. 2013. "Experience." In *Oxford English Dictionary*, 7th edition. Oxford: Oxford University Press.

Waites, Cheryl. 2009. "Building on Strengths: Intergenerational Practice with African American Families." *Social Work* 54 (3):278–87.

Wallace, Michele. 1979. *Black Macho and the Myth of the Superwoman*. New York: Dial.

Wallace, Maurice. 2007. "'I AM A MAN': Latent Doubt, Public Protest and the Anxious Construction of Black American Manhood." In *Ideology, Identity, and Assumptions* (Schomburg Studies on the Black Experience). Vol. 1, edited by Howard Dodson and Colin Palmer, 133–78. East Lansing: Michigan State University Press.

Washington, Booker T., ed. 2003 [1903]. *The Negro Problem: A Series of Articles by Representative American Negros of Today*. Amherst, MA: Humanity Books.

Weiss, Billie. 2007. "Fact Sheet: Gang Violence." The Violence Prevention Coalition of Greater Los Angeles. http://www.ph.ucla.edu/sciprc/pdf/GANG_VIOLENCE.pdf.

Weiss, Meira. 1997. "Signifying the Pandemics: Metaphors of AIDS, Cancer, and Heart Disease." *Medical Anthropology Quarterly* 11 (4):456–76.

Wentzer, Thomas. 2012. "The Meaning of Being." In *Routledge Companion to Phenomenology*, edited by Sebastian Luft and Søren Overgaard, 347–58. London: Routledge.

———. 2014. "'I Have Seen Konigsberg Burning': Philosophical Anthropology and the Responsiveness of Historical Experience." *Anthropological Theory* 14(1):27–48.

West, Cornel. 1996. "Black Strivings." In *The Future of the Race*, edited by Henry Gates Jr. and Cornel West, 53–112. New York: Knopf.

———. 2001 [1993]. *Race Matters*. Boston: Beacon Press.

———. 2008. *Hope on a Tightrope*. Carlsbad, CA: Hay House.

White, Hayden. 1980. "The Value of Narrativity in the Representation of Reality." In *On Narrative*, edited by W.J. Thomas Mitchell. Chicago: University of Chicago Press.

———. 1987. *The Content of the Form: Narrative Discourse and Historical Representation*. Baltimore: Johns Hopkins University Press.

———. 1999. *Figural Realism: Studies in the Mimesis Effect*. Baltimore: John Hopkins University Press.

White, Joseph, and James Cones. 1999. *Black Man Emerging: Facing the Past and Seizing a Future in America*. New York: Routledge.

Wiener, Margaret J. 2003. "Hidden Forces: Colonialism and the Politics of Magic in the Netherlands East Indies." In *Magic and Modernity: Interfaces of Revelation and Concealment*, edited by Birgit Meyer and Peter Pels. Stanford University Press.

Wiener, Margaret J. 2004. "Making Worlds through Religion, Science and Magic." *Anthropology News* 45(8):10–11.

Wikan, Unni. 1990. *Managing Turbulent Hearts: A Balinese Formula for Living*. Chicago: University of Chicago Press.

Willen, Sarah. 2010. "Darfur through a Shoah Lens: Sudanese Asylum Seekers, Unruly Biopolitical Dramas, and the Politics of Humanitarian Compassion in Israel. In *A Reader in Medical Anthropology: Theoretical Trajectories, Emergent Realities*, Vol. 15, edited by B.J. Good, M.M. Fischer, S.S. Willen, and M.J.D. Good, 505–21. New York: Wiley.

Willerslev, Rane, and Lotte Meinert. n.d.

Williams, Bernard. 1981. *Moral Luck: Philosophical Papers*. Cambridge: Cambridge University Press.

Williams, Melvin. 1974. *Community in a Black Pentecostal Church*. Prospect Heights, IL: Waveland.

Williams, Raymond. 1989. *Resources of Hope: Culture, Democracy, Socialism*. London: Verso.

Willis, Paul. 1981. *Learning to Labor: How Working Class Kids Get Working Class Jobs*. New York: Columbia University Press.

Willis, Tom (director). 2010. *Inside Bloods and Crips: L.A. Gangs*. National Geographic Channel. June 8. Documentary, 45:24 minutes. http://www.youtube.com/watch?v = zl3QhUHDM90.

Wilson, Sonja, and Margaret Miles. 2001. "Spirituality in African-American Mothers Coping with a Seriously Ill Infant." *Journal for Specialists in Pediatric Nursing* 6 (3):116–22.

Winch, Peter. 1958. *The Idea of a Social Science and Its Relation to Philosophy*. London: Routledge and Kegan Paul.

Wingard, Leah. 2007. "Constructing Time and Prioritizing Activities in Parent–Child Interaction." *Discourse and Society* 18 (1):75–91.

Wingood, Gina, Ralph DiClemente, Rick Crosby, Kathy Harrington, Susan Davies, and Edward Hook. 2002. "Gang Involvement and the Health of African American Female Adolescents." *Pediatrics* 110 (5):e57.

Wolcott, Victoria W. 1997. ""Bible, Bath and Broom": Nannie Helen Burrough's National Training School and African American Racial Uplift." *Journal of Women's History* 9 (1):88–110.

Woodard, Jennifer Bailey, and Teresa Mastin. 2005. "Black Womanhood: *Essence* and Its Treatment of Stereotypical Images of Black Women." *Journal of Black Studies* 36 (2):264–81.

von Wright, Georg Henrik. 1971. *Explanation and Understanding.* Ithaca, NY: Cornell University Press.

Yan, Yunxiang. 2011. "How Far Away Can We Move from Durkheim? Reflections on the New Anthropology of Morality." *Anthropology of This Century,* 2. http:aotcpress.com/articles/move-durkhein-reflections-anthropology-morality/.

Young, Allan. 1995. *The Harmony of Illusions: Inventing Posttraumatic Stress Disorder.* Princeton: Princeton University Press.

Zahavi, Dan. 2005. *Subjectivity and Selfhood: Investigating the First-Person Perspective.* Cambridge, MA: MIT Press.

Zigon, Jarrett. 2007. "Moral Breakdown and the Ethical Demand: A Theoretical Framework for an Anthropology of Moralities." *Anthropological Theory* 7 (2):131–50.

———. 2008. *Morality: An Anthropological Perspective.* Oxford: Berg.

———. 2009. "Within a Range of Possibilities: Morality and Ethics in Social Life." *Ethnos* 74 (2):251–76.

———. 2010. "Moral and Ethical Assemblages: A Response to Fassin and Stoczkowski." *Anthropological Theory* 10 (3):3–15.

———. 2011. *HIV Is God's Blessing: Rehabilitating Morality in Neoliberal Russia.* Berkeley: University of California Press.

Index

community: action as requiring, 82; deliberation about ethics, 119–121; the good life and, 10, 115–116; the moral self and, 40–41; and narrative re-envisioning, 87–89; the self as constructed via reference to, 22–25; suffering for, 25. See also family; intersubjectivity

compassion, 17, 84–85, 97, 170

Cones, James, 228n2(183)

Conner, Norma, 228n9(186)

Connolly, William, 54

courtroom, moral becoming as, 62–63, 70–72, 200, 224nn2–3(62)

Craven, Christa, 158–159

Crow people, 28

Crowell, Steven, 219–220n13

Csordas, Thomas J., 84, 224nn25,27(56)

cultural resources for transformation and critique: authoritative moral discourse critiques another, 186, 187–193; the black church as, 166–167, 191–201, 227n10(166); challenges from within a moral authority, 186, 193–197; children's verbal play, 92–96, 97–98; confession, 186; definition of, 53; home routines/rituals, 92–93, 97–98; indigenous sources of critique and hope, 199–200; primary resources for, 26–27, 186; the streets, 76–77, 79, 186, 187–193; third person perspective utilized, 186, 193–199, 200–201. See also family; moral laboratories

Das, Veena, 55, 77–78, 208, 223n17(49)

Dave, Naisargi N., 224–225n6(63)

Davis-Floyd, Robbie, 226n3(159)

de Certeau, Michel, 159

deontology, 37

Desjarlais, R.R., 44, 52, 224nn25–27(56)

Dray, W.H., 221–222n9(37)

Dreyfus, Hubert, xv–xvi, 222–223n16(49)

Du Bois, W.E. B, 176

Durkheim, Emile, 35, 223n19(55)

Edleson, Jeffrey L., 181

Edwards, Jeanette, 228n2(183)

Eller, Lucille, 228n9(186)

Elliot, Mary Horton, 227n11(166)

Ellison, Christopher, 228nn11,13(196,197)

Ellison, Ralph, 178

ethical and moral, as equivalent terms in text, 5

ethics, defined, 28

ethnography, and first person perspective, 41, 206

Eugene, Toinette M., 228n12(197)

events: as illustrating moral dilemmas and tasks, 8–9; and the three-fold present, 18

everyday life. See moral becoming; moral ordinary

evil, 11

existentialism, 36, 45

experiential givenness, 12–13

experimental (subjunctive) self, 123–125, 226n2(123); and the play of possible lives, 125–149

facticity, 9

family: flexibility of kinship arrangements, 6; and friendship, dialogue of, 90–92; illness shared by, 124–125; importance of, to African American community, 6; moral learning within, 39, 222nn11–12(39); narrative re-envisioning by, 88–89; raising "good" children as universal function of, 6. See also Superstrong Black Mother

Farran, Carol, 227n11(166)

Fassin, Didier, 11, 41, 51–52, 220n22(20)

Faubion, James D., 35, 41, 48–49, 63, 220–221n2(34), 220n23(26), 224–225nn1,6(62,63)

feminism, and connected vs. autonomous self, 39

first person perspective: as analytic starting point, 206; anthropology as eschewing, 43; as communal (see community; intersubjectivity); and daily rituals/routines of home care, 64–67; ethnography and, 41, 206; and experiential givenness, 13; and friendship, moral becoming via, 90–91; and ground projects and self as mutually constituting, 12–13; and locus of ethical agency, 47; and objects, subjectivity of, 49; phenomenology and, 12–14, 36–37, 56–57, 224n26(56); plural, 47, 66, 88, 205; and possibility, exploration of, 205–206; as relational, 204; and responsivity, 13; and significance of events, 22; and subjectivity, 14; temporality and, 18–19; "thick" version of the moral self and, 18–19, 38, 39, 83, 118, 205; third person perspective contrasted with, 12–14, 29, 200–201, 205, 219–220n13. See also first person virtue ethics

CPSIA information can be obtained
at www.ICGtesting.com
Printed in the USA
LVOW12s0842090318
569263LV00001B/3/P